Diagnostic Tests Toolkit

Matthew Thompson
Associate Professor, Department of Family Medicine
Oregon Health & Science University,
Portland, Oregon, USA
& Senior Clinical Scientist
Department of Primary Care Health Sciences
University of Oxford, Oxford, UK

Ann Van den Bruel
Academic Clinical Lecturer
Department of Primary Care Health Sciences
University of Oxford, Oxford, UK

SERIES EDITORS:

**Carl Heneghan, Rafael Perera
and Douglas Badenoch**

BMJ|Books

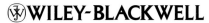

A John Wiley & Sons, Ltd., Publication

This edition first published 2012, © 2012 by John Wiley & Sons Ltd

BMJ Books is an imprint of BMJ Publishing Group Limited, used under licence by Blackwell Publishing which was acquired by John Wiley & Sons in February 2007. Blackwell's publishing programme has been merged with Wiley's global Scientific, Technical and Medical business to form Wiley-Blackwell.

Registered office: John Wiley & Sons, Ltd, The Atrium, Southern Gate, Chichester, West Sussex, PO19 8SQ, UK

Editorial offices: 9600 Garsington Road, Oxford, OX4 2DQ, UK
The Atrium, Southern Gate, Chichester, West Sussex, PO19 8SQ, UK
111 River Street, Hoboken, NJ 07030-5774, USA

For details of our global editorial offices, for customer services and for information about how to apply for permission to reuse the copyright material in this book please see our website at www.wiley.com/wiley-blackwell

A catalogue record for this book is available from the British Library.

Library of Congress Cataloging-in-Publication Data

Thompson, Matthew J.
    Diagnostic tests toolkit / Matthew Thompson, Ann Van den Bruel.
        p. ; cm. – (EBM toolkit series)
    Includes bibliographical references and index.
    ISBN-13: 978-0-4706-5758-4 (pbk. : alk. paper)
    ISBN-10: 0-470-65758-8 (pbk. : alk. paper)
    1. Diagnosis–Handbooks, manuals, etc. 2. Function tests
(Medicine)–Handbooks, manuals, etc. I. Van den Bruel, Ann. II. Title. III. Series: EBM toolkit series.
    [DNLM: 1. Diagnostic Techniques and Procedures–Handbooks. 2. Evidence-Based
Medicine–Handbooks. WB 39]
    RC71.T56 2011
    616.07'5–dc23

                                                                            2011020600

This book is published in the following electronic formats: ePDF 9781119951797; Wiley Online Library 9781119951827; ePub 9781119951803; mobi 9781119951810

Set in 7/9 pt Frutiger Light by Toppan Best-set Premedia Limited
Printed and bound in Malaysia by Vivar Printing Sdn Bhd

1 2012

Contents

Acknowledgements

This handbook was compiled by Matthew Thompson and Ann Van den Bruel based on teaching materials and workshops that we and other members of the Centre for Evidence-based Medicine have fine-tuned over a number of years for diagnostic tests. We particularly appreciate the input of the Toolkit Series Editors Carl Heneghan, Rafael Perera and Doug Badenoch. MT and AvdB thank their families for support in writing this book.

Introduction

This 'Toolkit' is designed as a summary and reminder of the key elements of practising evidence-based medicine (EBM), focusing on diagnostic studies and research questions. It has largely been adapted from resources developed at the Centre for Evidence-based Medicine. For more detailed coverage, you should refer to the further reading and references that we cite throughout.

The first page of each chapter presents a 'minimalist' checklist of the key points. Further sections within each chapter address these points in more detail and give additional background information. Ideally, you should just need to refer to the first page to get the basics, and delve into the further sections as required.

Definition of evidence-based medicine

Evidence-based medicine is the 'conscientious, explicit and judicious use of current best evidence in making decisions about individual patients'.

This means 'integrating individual clinical expertise with the best available external clinical evidence from systematic research and the patient's values and preferences' (Sackett et al. 1996).

We can summarize the EBM approach as a five-step model:

1. Asking answerable clinical questions.
2. Searching for the evidence.
3. Critically appraising the evidence for its validity and relevance.
4. Making a decision, by integrating the evidence with your clinical expertise and the patient's values.
5. Evaluating your performance.

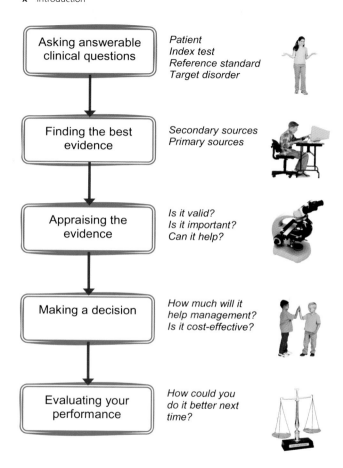

Asking answerable clinical questions

Patient
Index test
Reference standard
Target disorder

Finding the best evidence

Secondary sources
Primary sources

Appraising the evidence

Is it valid?
Is it important?
Can it help?

Making a decision

How much will it help management?
Is it cost-effective?

Evaluating your performance

How could you do it better next time?

Reference

Sackett DL, Rosenberg WMC, Gray JAM, et al. Evidence based medicine: what it is and what it isn't. *BMJ* 1996;**312**:71–2.

CHAPTER 1

Diagnosis in evidence-based medicine

Diagnosis and screening

The main goal of diagnostic tests is to identify the likely cause of an illness in patients presenting with clinical features, and to direct subsequent treatment. Diagnostic tests often have other uses, such as giving information about the prognosis of a condition, or monitoring patients during the course of an illness. Screening tests, in contrast, are usually used in otherwise healthy individuals to identify those who have an illness that has not yet caused any symptoms or signs.

Some diagnostic and screening tests have been used for hundreds (or even thousands of years), such as physical examination. Others have emerged as our understanding of disease processes has increased, coupled with advances in science and technology. Individuals, clinicians and health-care systems are now faced with a dazzling variety of different tests, ranging from simple point-of-care blood tests to complex imaging systems.

Unfortunately, few diagnostic tests are 100% accurate. Similar to treatments, diagnostic tests need to be evaluated in rigorous research. However, studies of diagnostic tests are often reported poorly, and many clinicians have difficulty understanding the results of diagnostic tests. Indeed a survey of 300 physicians in the USA found that 95% did not use numeric measures of diagnostic accuracy (sensitivity, specificity, likelihood ratios), but rather relied on their experience of tests in their patients and setting. This suggests that understanding even these diagnostic accuracy measures is difficult for most clinicians, let alone considering other outcomes of diagnostic tests. The dangers with this approach are that clinicians' biases can become entrenched in practice (some of which may be correct and some incorrect), and it becomes difficult to incorporate new tests or new diagnostic information into practice.

Evidence-based medicine emphasizes clinical research and a critical appraisal of that research, rather than unsystematic clinical experience or opinion. This does not mean that clinical experience and an understanding of the underlying pathophysiology have become redundant. In fact, especially in diagnosis, the clinical instinct or 'gut feeling' that is acquired

Diagnostic Tests Toolkit, First Edition. Matthew Thompson, Ann Van den Bruel.
© 2012 John Wiley & Sons, Ltd. Published 2012 by John Wiley & Sons, Ltd.

through experience is an important diagnostic tool. Evidence-based diagnosis seeks to combine clinical expertise with the best available evidence, while taking into account patient preferences.

Roles of diagnostic tests in health care

Role	Description	Examples
Confirming or excluding a diagnosis	Used to confirm ('rule in') or exclude ('rule out') particular diagnoses. Most tests will be better at one than the other. May vary between different clinical settings/different spectrum of disease	Normal blood pressure measurement to exclude hypertension Raised cardiac troponins to confirm cardiac ischaemia
Triage	An initial test in a clinical pathway, which usually determines the need for further (usually more invasive) testing. Ideal triage test is usually fairly rapid, and should not miss any patients (i.e. minimize false negatives)	Blood pressure and heart rate in initial triage of patients with multiple trauma to identify those with possible shock D-Dimer to screen for presence of pulmonary embolism in patients who have shortness of breath
Monitoring	Tests that are repeated at periodic intervals in patients with chronic conditions, or in those receiving certain treatments, in order to assess efficacy of interventions, disease progression or need for changes in treatment	Glycated haemoglobin (HbA1c) to monitor glucose control in patients with diabetes Anticoagulation tests for patients taking oral anticoagulants (warfarin) Viral load and CD4 cell counts in patients with HIV infection
Prognosis	Provides information on disease course or progression, and individual response to treatment	CT scans in patients with known ovarian cancer to determine the stage
Screening	Detecting conditions or risk factors for conditions in people who are apparently asymptomatic.	Mammography screening for breast cancer Cholesterol testing to detect people at greater risk of cardiovascular disease

Different types of diagnostic tests

In clinical practice, we use different types of tests, each with their own strengths and weaknesses. In general, tests that are readily available and painless are used in unselected patient groups (e.g. primary care), whereas tests with increasing level of invasiveness, costs and risks of harmful side effects are used in more highly selected patient populations (e.g. tertiary care hospital settings).

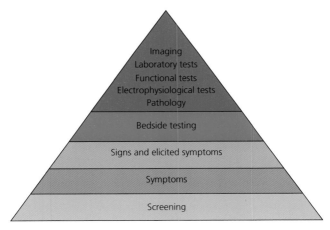

Imaging
Laboratory tests
Functional tests
Electrophysiological tests
Pathology

Bedside testing

Signs and elicited symptoms

Symptoms

Screening

Figure 1.1

Screening

Screening is performed in individuals who do not currently have any symptoms or clinical signs to suggest the target condition. It is used in unselected target populations, who may be defined by age (e.g. screening for hypertension in elderly people) or gender (e.g. mammography in women), or other 'risk factors'. The rationale and pitfalls of screening are discussed in Chapter 9.

Symptoms

In general, patients seek medical attention because they are experiencing certain symptoms. They might have a cough that is worrisome or feel pain. These symptoms can be used as diagnostic tests, and therefore have a diagnostic value for a particular target disorder. For example, a patient presenting to a clinician complaining of crushing central chest pain might be suspected of having a heart attack (myocardial infarction).

Signs and elicited symptoms

Symptoms and physical signs assessed during physical examination may have a different diagnostic value to those spontaneously reported by a patient. For example, certain symptoms that are commonly elicited from patients who are complaining of chest pain (such as worsening with exertion or spreading to the left shoulder) may increase the likelihood of a myocardial infarction. In addition, clinicians may observe physical abnormalities such as paleness or sweating, or an irregular pulse rate. Some physical signs are measures of physiological variables, such as blood pressure or fever. Developing clinical expertise involves not only learning how to elicit these clinical features, but also understanding their diagnostic value, including how reliable or repeatable they are (see Chapter 2 on inter- and intraobserver agreement).

Bedside or point-of-care testing

Many diagnostic tests are now available as point of care tests. These include tests on samples of urine (e.g. pregnancy tests), fingerstick drops of blood (e.g. glucose levels), or microbiological swabs (e.g. rapid antigen test for Group A streptococci in throat swabs). These tests are typically automated or simple to perform. Many tests that formerly required larger volumes of blood, or laboratory equipment, are now performed in real time during patient consultations. Point of care tests may be all that are required to exclude a condition (e.g. a negative throat strep test would usually exclude streptococcal tonsillitis) or confirm a condition (e.g. a positive urine pregnancy test).

Laboratory tests

A vast number of more complex tests are typically performed only in laboratory or hospital settings, and involve a higher degree of skill to perform or interpret. These include the specialties of biochemistry, haematology, microbiology, radiology and pathology. Some involve no or minimal invasiveness (e.g. many blood tests, ultrasonography), whereas others may require more invasive procedures (e.g. coronary angiography, liver biopsy).

Additional types of diagnostic tests that are available only in hospital (or hospital outpatient) settings include many types of endoscopy, as well as functional tests (e.g. exercise ECG treadmill tests).

Basic structure of studies of diagnostic tests

The aim of diagnostic accuracy studies is usually to find out how well a test performs at ruling in (confirming) or ruling out (excluding) a clinical condition. This means that the results of a new test (the index test) are compared with the results of the reference standard (or 'gold standard'). The reference standard is the test that is considered to be best at diagnosing the target condition in which you are interested.

Diagnostic test studies generally all share the same basic structure: a series of patients (or study participants) are selected; they all receive the index test, followed by the reference standard. Finally the results of the index test and reference standard are compared with each other.

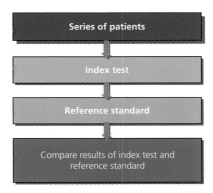

Figure 1.2

Further reading

Irwig L, Bossuyt PM, Glasziou P et al. Designing studies to ensure that estimates of test accuracy are transferable. *BMJ* 2002;**324**:669–71.

Knottnerus JA. *The Evidence Base of Clinical Diagnosis*. London: BMJ Books, 2002.

Knottnerus JA, Muris JW. Assessment of the accuracy of diagnostic tests: the cross-sectional study. *J Clin Epidemiol* 2003;**56**:1118–28.

Sackett DL, Haynes RB. The architecture of diagnostic research. *BMJ* 2002;**324**:539–41.

CHAPTER 2
Evaluating new diagnostic tests

WHAT ARE THE KEY STEPS?
1. Technical accuracy
'Can it work?'
2. Place in the clinical pathway
'Where does the test fit in the existing clinical pathway?'
3. Ability of the test to diagnose or exclude the target condition
'Does it work in patients?'
4. The effect of the test on patient outcomes
'Are patients better off?'
5. Cost-effectiveness
'Is it worth the cost'?

New tests are continually being developed, and tests that are already in use are often part of ongoing evaluation studies. New diagnostic devices are subject to regulatory approval, but this is highly variable between countries. In general, new diagnostic devices can be approved and marketed without having to show that they improve clinical outcomes – unlike new medications where this is a standard part of approval.

As a result, individual clinicians, hospitals and health-care systems often need to evaluate new tests. Many countries devote considerable resources to assess and compare new and emerging health technologies, including numerous health technology assessment (HTA) or comparative effectiveness organisations, horizon scanning groups, as well as many professional societies and private sector health insurers or health maintenance organisations.

Typically, diagnostic tests are judged by their ability to diagnose or exclude an illness or target condition. However, other aspects of a new test such as impact on patient outcome or value for money may be equally important. A number of different frameworks have been proposed to evaluate new diagnostic tests. These typically include five aspects, as shown in the table:

1. Technical accuracy
2. Place in the clinical pathway
3. Diagnostic accuracy
4. Effect on patient outcome
5. Cost-effectiveness.

Diagnostic Tests Toolkit, First Edition. Matthew Thompson, Ann Van den Bruel.
© 2012 John Wiley & Sons, Ltd. Published 2012 by John Wiley & Sons, Ltd.

Information type	Question	Output	Study designs
Technical accuracy	Is the test reliable under standardized, artificial conditions?	Analytical sensitivity and specificity Reproducibility, i.e. accuracy, precision and observer variation	Accuracy studies using standardized material, such as bloodbank samples
Place in clinical pathway	Where does the new test fit in existing clinical pathways?	Identification of current diagnostic pathway for a condition. Problems with current pathway (e.g. time, costs, side effects of tests) Opportunities for new test to improve clinical outcomes	Reviews of existing diagnostic pathways Descriptions of attributes of new tests
Diagnostic accuracy	How good is this test at confirming or excluding a target condition?	Sensitivity and specificity, likelihood ratios, area under the curve	Diagnostic accuracy studies including real patients, comparing the new test with a reference standard
Impact on patient outcome	After introducing this test to the clinical pathway, do patients fare better?	Mortality, morbidity, functional status, quality of life	Randomized controlled trials Clinical non-randomized trials Before-after studies
Cost-effectiveness	Is this test good value for money?	Cost per life-year gained, cost per quality-adjusted life-year	Economic modelling

All of these ask different questions, provide different pieces of information about a test, and need different study designs to address them. Ideally, a new test would be assessed against each of these in turn.

Technical accuracy ('Can it work?')

Does it measure what it is meant to?

Before applying a test to real patients, the test needs to be technically sound. This refers to the test's ability to measure the parameter or quantity of interest under standardized conditions, i.e. outside clinical practice. Although this is the initial step in evaluating a new test, finding out about a test's technical accuracy is not always straightforward. Not all tests are evaluated on these aspects. For many clinical diagnostic tests such as symptoms and examination signs, this is lacking. In addition, evidence on the reproducibility of tests that are already marketed may not be available in the public domain.

For example, laboratory tests will be evaluated on artificial samples that contain a known quantity of the parameter of interest. Other examples include the use of 'phantoms', which are devices that simulate part of the human body, e.g. an artificial thorax in evaluating the ability of PET (positron emission tomography) scans to detect pulmonary nodules, or devices that simulate body temperature that are used to assess thermometers. Analytical sensitivity measures whether the test can detect a known quantity of the parameter of interest. Analytical specificity can be determined by assessing samples that do not contain the parameter of interest but rather a *different* parameter that might lead to a false-positive result.

Is it reproducible?

In addition to the test's ability to measure the parameter of interest, it is important to assess its reproducibility (also called precision). Will the test produce the same result on different occasions or when interpreted by different observers? Reproducibility depends on analytical variability and observer variation.

Analytical variability consists of *inaccuracy*, which is a systematic error, and *imprecision*, which is a random error. The difference between the two is illustrated by the targets from a shooting range shown in Figure 2.1 – each spot represents one bullet hole. The first 'target' shows a test that is very precise, i.e. all the shots end up hitting the target in pretty much the same spot, but it is way off the centre bull's eye (i.e. it is not accurate). The second target shows a test that is accurate (if you could 'average' all the shots, this average would be close to the bull's eye) but not precise (the shots are all

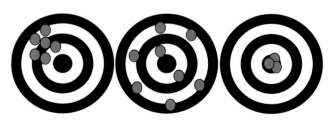

Precise, but not accurate

Accurate, but not precise

Precise and accurate

Figure 2.1

scattered around). The third target shows a test that is both accurate (all the shots hit the bull's eye) and precise (all the shots give the same result).

The second aspect of reproducibility is *observer variation*. Observer variation consists of interobserver variation and intraobserver variation.

Interobserver variation refers to the situation where two observers interpret the same test, and assesses the extent to which they agree or disagree about the result.

Intraobserver variation refers to the situation where the same observer interprets the same test on two different occasions.

This is illustrated by Figure 2.2. Let us say that a patient has a hearing test performed by two different audiologists (observer 1 and observer 2) on two different days. The level of agreement in the results of the hearing test that observer 1 obtains on day 1 and day 2 is the intraobserver variation. The difference in results of the hearing tests that observer 1 and observer 2 obtain on the same day is the interobserver variation.

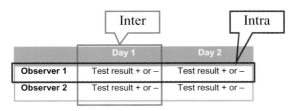

Figure 2.2

Place in the clinical pathway ('Where does the test fit in the existing clinical pathway?')

New tests can have many different potential roles, and it is important to identify what the role of the new test is expected to be in clinical practice. New diagnostic tests can have three main types of role in clinical pathways – they can replace another test, or act as a triage or an add-on test. These roles are not exclusive; some tests can have more than one role for different target conditions.

The intended role will define what type of study you need to assess whether the test will perform well in that role, and what results you need to look for.

Role of test	Description	Example	Most efficient study designs
Replacement	New test may be more accurate, easier, less painful or invasive, less costly, faster	Pulse oximetry instead of arterial blood gas for assessing severity of pneumonia	Paired study: patients tested with new test, existing test and reference standard Randomized trial: allocated to either existing OR new test, then all get the reference standard
Triage	New test to be used before an existing test, and results used to direct the need for further testing. This might lead to more patients needing further tests, or fewer patients needing the further tests	Ottawa ankle clinical prediction rule used to triage patients presenting with ankle injuries to decide who needs an ankle radiograph	Paired study: patients all get the triage test, existing test and reference standard Limited verification: do the reference standard only in those patients who have a negative result on the triage test but positive on the existing test
Add-on	New test will be used after the existing test or testing pathway, perhaps in a subgroup of patients	Using exercise ECG tests in patients who have negative resting ECG to identify those with ischaemic heart disease	Paired study or randomized trial may be inefficient. Could limit study to patients who are negative at end of existing testing pathway, then do the new add-on test and verify with reference standard

Ability of the test to diagnose or exclude the target condition ('Does it work in patients?')

The ability of a test to detect or rule out a condition of interest is called diagnostic accuracy or clinical validity. This includes the key measures of sensitivity, specificity, predictive values and likelihood ratios, which are provided by diagnostic accuracy studies. We discuss the interpretation of these measures in much greater detail in Chapter 7. There are several different study designs that could be used (see also table).

Cross-sectional cohort study

The prototype of a diagnostic study is a cross-sectional study, in which a cohort of individuals is assembled based on some suspicion or possibility of the target disorder. The cohort of patients is selected from a representative population that share some characteristic, e.g. clinical presentation, age. Both index test and reference standard are applied to them all and in every patient compared with each other (see Chapter 6).

Nested case–control study

A typical case–control study identifies people with a disease (i.e. cases) and a sample without the disease from the population (i.e. controls). The index test is then applied to each of them.

The main problem with this type of case–control study is that it is difficult to make sure that the cases and controls are representative of the overall population. Cases and controls have been subject to different work-ups, referrals etc., which leads to biased estimates of test accuracy. In addition, the cases and controls are often at the extreme ends of the spectrum of disease. You might compare this to a machine that has to separate light colours from dark colours in a pile of laundry. If all items of clothing in the laundry pile are either black or white, it will not be difficult for the test to separate these two groups. However, when the machine is trying to separate out different hues of grey rather than black from white (as is the case with most of our laundry!), then the machine's diagnostic accuracy may be much worse.

A nested case–control study, on the other hand, selects cases and controls from the same source population that has a known sample size, and have all had the same work-up (e.g. all presenting to an emergency department with chest pain). This means that all had the same reference standard, and cases and controls represent the entire spectrum of disease. Nested case–control studies can sometimes be more efficient than a full cohort study, particularly when an index test is difficult, costly or invasive. Diagnostic accuracies estimated in these types of studies are not likely to be different to a full cohort.

Paired study

The new test and existing test are performed in all study participants, and the results are compared with the reference standard that is also performed in all participants. In effect, this is an extension of the cross-sectional cohort study.

Randomized study

Patients are randomly allocated to receive either the new test or the existing test (or testing strategy), and they all have the reference standard. All patients are followed long enough not only to compare the new and existing tests to the reference standard, but also to assess any other differences in the new and existing tests. These might include side effects or other downstream consequences because of differences in who does and who does not receive treatment. This type of study is particularly useful for assessing the impacts of the decisions taken as a result of the diagnostic test, but can be difficult and expensive to conduct.

Indirect comparisons

The new test is performed in one group of patients (e.g. in one clinic), and compared with results of the existing test performed in a different population (e.g. a different clinic). This is subject to variations in the patients, selection and reference standard. Another type of study design in this category would be a before–after study, where diagnoses or processes before a new test or testing strategy are compared with the results *after* a new test or testing strategy has been implemented. These studies are all prone to bias.

The effect of the test on patient outcomes ('Are patients better off?')

Main outcomes of tests

The primary goal of a new test is to improve health outcomes of patients, e.g. how long they live, their level of function or disability. This is also called clinical utility. Apart from some rare clinical scenarios, the test *itself* does not improve health. The test has to enable the clinician and patient to take a different action than he or she did before having the test result. This is usually a change in the treatment plan to one that is more appropriate based on the result of the test. The patient then has to agree, and adhere, to the new treatment. Only then can the effects of the diagnostic test on patient outcome be assessed. This is one reason why diagnostic tests in themselves may have little effect on patient outcomes, and it is usually challenging to demonstrate a causal link between testing and clinical outcome.

Other test outcomes

Diagnostic tests can have effects on many other patient outcomes, such as their emotions, social functioning, cognition and behaviour.

Effects of testing	What this means	Effects on health
Emotional	Test causes harmful or beneficial changes in levels of anxiety, depression, stress, psychological wellbeing	Increased anxiety and stress occurring after a positive test on screening that has not been confirmed with a reference standard Reassurance and improved overall wellbeing after a negative test
Social	Effects of testing on social roles, social functions, sexual relationships, social relationships	Social isolation and stigmatization after a positive test Problems with employment or insurance coverage Genetic testing results may cause guilt about passing on a genetic predisposition
Cognitive	Patients' beliefs, perceptions and understanding about the test result and the condition	May understand disease better – what causes it, how long it lasts etc. – or affect adherence to therapy
Behavioural	The combinations of emotional, social and cognitive effects can affect patient behaviour. Positive and negative tests can prompt change in behaviour	Adherence to clinical intervention may be increased or decreased Greater or less engagement with other health-related behaviours, e.g. increased exercise after having cholesterol measured Perceptions of risks from screening and repeated screening

In some cases these additional 'secondary' outcomes may be equally or even more important than the main outcomes. One reason why it is important to consider the additional outcomes of diagnostic tests is because they have the potential to both augment and negate the effects on the primary outcome. For example, a test that results in a very large improvement in mortality or morbidity may be tolerated even though it causes a lot of distress. On the other hand, a test that offers little in terms of improving clinical outcomes may still be beneficial if it is associated with less anxiety, e.g. a rapid point-of-care HIV test may be preferable to a laboratory test taking several days. When assessing a new test, all these outcomes should be used to weigh up its benefits (e.g. improved quality of life, avoiding other tests, longer or better life) and harms (e.g. pain, risks, costs, side effects).

One reason why it is important to be aware of the many different aspects of the outcomes of diagnostic studies is so that studies can be designed to evaluate the test as fully as possible, taking all these into account. Studies that look only at effects on clinical outcome or effects on social outcomes are not going to be adequate to provide a true assessment of the effects of a test. In general it is important for studies of diagnostic tests to not only measure clinical outcomes, but also use various tools and measures of emotional, social, cognitive and behavioural outcomes. Quality-of-life measures go some way towards doing this, but other tools can be used as well.

Finally, some tests have a very narrow diagnostic scope (e.g. urine pregnancy tests), whereas others have a much wider range of conditions for which they may be valuable. For example, a chest radiograph can be used to investigate the presence or absence of pneumonia in an adult but may also be valuable to examine cardiac conditions (e.g. heart failure, cardiomegaly), gastroenterology (e.g. hiatus hernia) and bony conditions (e.g. fractures, bone density).

Cost-effectiveness ('Is it worth the cost?')

Evaluating the economic impacts of new tests on individuals, health-care systems or even countries is a final step in the evaluation process. There are several types of analysis that can be used. In general there are far fewer studies on economic impacts of tests than there are for other aspects of the evaluation of new tests.

Type of analysis	What it measures	Examples
Cost minimization analysis	What is the least costly test among several alternatives that have the same outcome?	The cost per test of point-of-care glucose tests compared with central laboratory glucose tests
Cost-effectiveness and cost utility analysis	Compares different tests in terms of money for health outcomes. Presents results as the costs per life saved, case prevented or quality-adjusted life-year (QALY)	Cost-effectiveness of screening for colon cancer using faecal occult blood test in terms of cost per QALY
Cost–benefit analysis	Compares the costs and benefits of a test, both of which are measured in monetary units	Net cost–benefit ratio of a new mammography imaging technique
Budget impact analysis	Estimates the financial impacts of adopting a new test in a given clinical setting or population	The costs of operating budget and capital expenditure of adopting and using a new test

Further reading

Bossuyt PM, McCaffery K. Additional patient outcomes and pathways in evaluations of testing. *Med Decis Making* 2009;**29**:E20–8.

Bossuyt PM, Irwig L, Craig J, Glasziou P. Comparative accuracy: assessing new tests against existing diagnostic pathways. *BMJ* 2006;**332**:1089–92.

Lijmer JG, Leeflang M, Bossuyt PM. Proposals for a phased evaluation of medical tests. *Med Decis Making* 2009;**29**:E13–21.

Newman-Toker DE, Pronovost PJ. Diagnostic errors – the next frontier for patient safety. *JAMA* 2009;**301**:1060–2.

Van den Bruel A, Cleemput I, Aertgeerts B, Ramaekers D, Buntinx F. The evaluation of diagnostic tests: evidence on technical and diagnostic accuracy, impact on patient outcome and cost-effectiveness is needed. *J Clin Epidemiol* 2007;**60**:1116–22.

CHAPTER 3
Asking an answerable clinical question

WHAT ARE THE KEY STEPS?
1. Define a precise clinical question and the information that you need to answer that question
2. Find the best available evidence by searching the literature
3. Assess its validity
4. Extract the clinical message
5. Evaluate the applicability to your patient, taking into account their values and preferences

---

Defining a clinical question for diagnostic tests – PIRT

Here are the four elements that are most useful for formulating an answerable clinical question about a diagnostic test's accuracy:
1. Patient/Problem
2. Index test
3. Reference standard
4. Target condition.

PIRT element	Tips	Specific example
Patient	'How would I describe a group of patients similar to mine?'	'In women aged 50 years or older and presenting with chest pain to their family doctor . . . '
Index test	'Which test am I considering?'	'. . . what is the diagnostic value of an exercise ECG stress test . . . '
Reference standard	'What is the reference standard considered to be ideal to diagnose the target disorder?'	'. . . compared with coronary angiography . . . '
Target condition	'Which diagnosis do I want to either rule in or rule out?'	'. . . for the diagnosis of symptomatic coronary artery disease?'

Diagnostic Tests Toolkit, First Edition. Matthew Thompson, Ann Van den Bruel.
© 2012 John Wiley & Sons, Ltd. Published 2012 by John Wiley & Sons, Ltd.

Although it can seem fairly straightforward and it is tempting to skip this step, it is absolutely vital to get this right. First, the terms that you identify from this process will form the basis of your search of the literature for the best evidence. Second, the question will act as your guide when you come to assess the relevance of the literature that you identify.

Patient/Problem

Describe your patients in terms of their presenting problem. How do they present clinically? The health-care setting is important, because diagnostic tests may have different values in different settings (e.g. primary or secondary care). Adding more details such as age or gender will focus your question and can help you later on in deciding whether the evidence is applicable to your specific question. However, you have to use some judgement because, if you are too specific, it can sometimes limit the evidence that you find.

Index test

This is the test that you are considering, the diagnostic value of which you would like to know. Again, you may want to add details if you want to focus your question, e.g. some tests such as the inflammatory marker C-reactive protein can be used as both a typical laboratory blood test and a point-of-care test on a drop of blood.

Reference standard

This is the test that is currently considered the ideal test ('gold standard') for diagnosing the target condition. In general, the reference standard is more invasive, takes longer or is more expensive than the index test. However, in many conditions there is no 'perfect' reference standard (or, at least, none that is feasible) and we sometimes have to make do with a less than ideal reference standard. Some reference standards consist of a series of tests, a clinical review panel or simply clinical follow-up.

Target condition

This is the illness or condition that you would like to diagnose (or exclude) in your patient. This may be an illness, such as myocardial infarction or femur fracture, but may also be a condition not necessarily considered an illness (but it may cause an illness later on), e.g. carotid artery stenosis.

Further reading

Knottnerus JA, van Weel C, Muris JW. Evaluation of diagnostic procedures. *BMJ* 2002;**324**:477–80.

Richardson WS, Wilson MC, Nishikawa J, Hayward RS. The well-built clinical question: a key to evidence-based decisions. *ACP J Club* 1995;**123**:A12–13.

CHAPTER 4

Finding the evidence: how to get the most from your searching

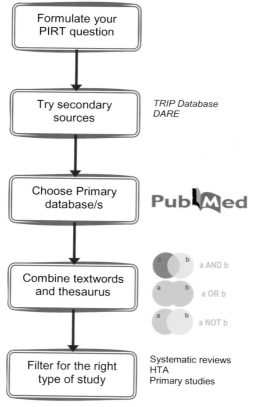

Figure 4.1

Diagnostic Tests Toolkit, First Edition. Matthew Thompson, Ann Van den Bruel.
© 2012 John Wiley & Sons, Ltd. Published 2012 by John Wiley & Sons, Ltd.

To use your time as efficiently as possible, start looking for answers by searching for secondary sources (e.g. evidence syntheses or systematic reviews) and go to primary sources only if you don't find the information that you are looking for in secondary sources.

Secondary sources for diagnostic questions include TRIP, DARE, the Cochrane Library (now also publishing diagnostic systematic reviews), Medion, Bandolier, ACP Journal Club (see table). Bookmark some of these in your browser; the more you use them the easier it will become to find what you need quickly.

Guidelines can be a useful source too, if they are developed using sound methods and your question has more to do with finding the best option among several than with finding precise information on one particular test. Guidelines do need to be adapted to your particular context, so guidance from other countries or domains may not always be applicable to your situation. Some guidelines are produced with a particular audience in mind, so they may not always be objective or comprehensive.

Secondary sources		
Systematic reviews	Review of all available evidence	DARE, the Cochrane Database of Systematic Reviews, Medion, Medline or Embase using a search filter such as Clinical Queries
Health technology assessments	Review of all available evidence including economic evaluation and organisational aspects	INAHTA, DARE, EUnetHTA
Evidence-based summaries	Reviews of the evidence around a specific clinical topic	BMJ Clinical Evidence, AHRQ Effective Health Care summaries
Structured abstracts	Appraisals of important clinical papers	ACP Journal Club, various 'journal watch' sources
Guidelines	Comprehensive guidance on the management of a target condition	NICE, SIGN, AHRQ National Guideline Clearinghouse

Primary sources include the major databases, such as Medline and Embase, but also CINAHL, PEDRO, PsycLit, etc. Searching these databases can be very time-consuming, so make sure that you focus your question well. Another difficulty of these sources is access to the information: unless you can access many journals electronically through your institution, finding the abstract but not the full text of the paper can be very frustrating!

Combine textwords and thesaurus

You can then combine terms from your well-formulated *PIRT* question (*patient – index test – reference standard – target condition*) with AND, OR, NOT. Using the same example as above, you can combine thesaurus terms (in PubMed they are called MeSH terms – Medical Subject Headings).

Element	Specific example	Search terms for MEDLINE (via PubMed)
Patient/problem	'In women aged 50 years or older and presenting with chest pain to their family doctor . . . '	'Chest Pain'[Mesh]
Index test	'. . . what is the diagnostic value of the treadmill ECG exercise stress test . . . '	'Exercise Test'[Mesh]
Reference standard	'. . . compared with coronary angiography . . . '	'Coronary Angiography'[Mesh]
Target condition	'. . . for the diagnosis of coronary artery disease?'	'Coronary Artery Disease'[Mesh]

What to do when you find *too few studies*?
- Use less specific terms, e.g. use 'Coronary Disease'[MeSH] instead of 'Coronary Artery Disease'[MeSH].
- Eliminate some terms, e.g. the terms referring to the reference standard.
- Use text words and find as many synonyms for the term as you can, e.g. exercise test OR stress test OR treadmill test.
- You can also truncate your terms and use wildcards, e.g. in PubMed, exercise test* will search for *exercise test, exercise tests* and *exercise testing*.

What to do when you find *too many studies*?
- Be more specific in the terms that you have used, e.g. replace 'Coronary Disease'[MeSH] by 'Coronary Artery Disease'[MeSH].
- Try to add more details, e.g. age or gender.
- Restrict your search to a specific type of study, such as diagnostic accuracy studies with a search filter (see below).
- Do not use text words or try to be more specific with those that you do want to use.

Search filters for diagnostic accuracy studies

Some databases offer a built-in search that filters your results so that it identifies only certain types of study designs, e.g. studies about diagnosis or systematic reviews. These filters can be used to focus your search, but the effect can be variable depending on the other terms that you are using. Filters will reduce the number of 'hits', i.e. articles that the search finds, at the expense of missing out studies that are potentially relevant. Many diagnostic search filters do not have very good sensitivity, unlike the search filters used in searches for randomized trials of interventions, which typically offer equally high specificity and sensitivity.

A well-known example is the Clinical Queries button in PubMed to search Medline, which works well in reducing the number needed to read while not missing too many studies. More filters are available from the published literature (see Further reading).

	Diagnostic accuracy studies	**Randomized controlled trials**
Sensitive filter	Sensitivity 98%, Specificity 74%	Sensitivity 99%, Specificity 70%
	(sensitiv*[Title/Abstract] OR sensitivity and specificity[MeSH Terms] OR diagnos*[Title/Abstract] OR diagnosis[MeSH:noexp] OR diagnostic*[MeSH:noexp] OR diagnosis, differential[MeSH:noexp] OR diagnosis[Subheading:noexp])	((clinical[Title/Abstract] AND trial[Title/Abstract]) OR clinical trials[MeSH Terms] OR clinical trial[Publication Type] OR random*[Title/Abstract] OR random allocation[MeSH Terms] OR therapeutic use[MeSH Subheading])
Specific filter	Sensitivity 64% Specificity 98% or specificity[Title/Abstract]	Sensitivity 93% Specificity 97% (randomized controlled trial[Publication Type] OR (randomized[Title/Abstract] AND controlled[Title/Abstract] AND trial[Title/Abstract])

Further reading

Bachmann LM, Coray R, Estermann P, Ter Riet G. Identifying diagnostic studies in MEDLINE: reducing the number needed to read. *J Am Med Inform Assoc* 2002;**9**:653–8.

Haynes RB, Wilczynski NL. Optimal search strategies for retrieving scientifically strong studies of diagnosis from Medline: analytical survey. *BMJ* 2004;**328**:1040.

Kastner M, Wilczynski NL, McKibbon AK, Garg AX, Haynes RB. Diagnostic test systematic reviews: bibliographic search filters ('Clinical Queries') for diagnostic accuracy studies perform well. *J Clin Epidemiol* 2009;**62**:974–81.

Wilczynski NL, Haynes RB, Hedges Team. EMBASE search strategies for identifying methodologically sound diagnostic studies for use by clinicians and researchers. *BMC Med* 2005;**3**:7.

CHAPTER 5

Selecting relevant studies

Once you have done your search, you need to select the studies that are the most relevant and the most valid. A study might be perfectly believable (i.e. internally valid), but just not relevant (or generalisable) to your particular setting. In contrast you might find a study that appears highly relevant to your setting, but it is just not valid.

WHAT ARE THE KEY STEPS?
1. Is the study relevant?
2. Is it true – do I believe it?

Selecting relevant studies

Go back to your well-formulated question and be as selective as you can. Is the study's research question sufficiently similar to your question? If the research study is too different from the one in which you are interested, you might want to go back and search again. If your search did not yield many studies, you may need to drop some details and use studies that are perhaps less directly applicable to your question.

Sources of variability	Questions to ask
Research question	How closely does it match my question?
Patients or participants	Are the patients in the study comparable to my patients? Consider their demographics, disease severity, prevalence of target condition, clinical setting
Index test	Is the index test similar to the one that I intend to use? Has it been described adequately so that it can be reproduced? Is it feasible or affordable to do it in my setting?
Reference standard	Is the reference standard truly the reference standard for this target condition? Is there a new reference standard available now? Has it been described adequately?
Target condition	Is the target condition the same as the one that I am interested in?

Diagnostic Tests Toolkit, First Edition. Matthew Thompson, Ann Van den Bruel.
© 2012 John Wiley & Sons, Ltd. Published 2012 by John Wiley & Sons, Ltd.

Assessing validity

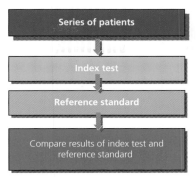

To assess validity keep in mind the basic structure of a diagnostic study.

A series of patients (or study subjects) is selected, they all get the index test, followed by the reference standard. Finally the results of the index test and reference standard are compared with each other.

Figure 5.1

What is the difference between *bias* and *variability* in diagnostic studies?

Variability occurs when there are differences in the way that a diagnostic study is carried out. This does not cause biased (or incorrect) estimates of the test performance, but may limit the generalisability of the study results. For example, a treadmill exercise test may have different diagnostic value in women and men. Depending on the composition of the patient population, studies may find different results. These are due not to bias, but to differences in the patient population.

   Bias occurs when there are problems ('defects') in either the design of a study or how it is carried out. This may result in estimates of the performance of a test that are not true (or at least not completely correct). Using the treadmill exercise test again as an example, results would be biased if the study included healthy students as controls for patients with definite coronary artery disease. In this situation, the diagnostic value of the test is artificially inflated, and does not reflect its value in a real clinical situation.

The 'ideal' diagnostic study

Key features to look for in the methods section are shown in the table.

Sources of internal validity	Questions to ask	What is ideal?
Selection of patients or participants	Was there an appropriate spectrum of patients selected?	The test should be performed on a group of patients similar to those in whom it will be applied in the real world
Index test	Was the reference standard performed on all patients?	All patients get the index test
Reference standard	Is the same reference test performed in all patients, regardless of the results of the index test? Is the reference test an objective test or more subjective?	All patients get the reference standard test. The reference standard is independent of the index test, and is objective
Comparison of index and reference test	Was there an independent, blind or objective comparison with the reference standard?	The investigator who is comparing the results of the index and reference tests should be blinded, i.e. they do not know the results of the other test

Flow charts of patients

Flow charts of patients display how many patients were eligible for the study, how many were actually recruited, how many received the index test, how many received the reference standard, etc. In addition, the number of true and false positives and true and false negatives are displayed.

The STARD (STAndards for the Reporting of Diagnostic accuracy studies) guidelines for reporting studies of diagnostic accuracy (see inside covers) recommend using flow charts in reports of primary diagnostic studies (Figure 5.2), because they are an easy way to understand the flow of patients through a study and to assess potential problems with selection bias, and they also present the results of the index test so that sensitivity and specificity can be derived. The STARD website has this information available at www.stard-statement.org.

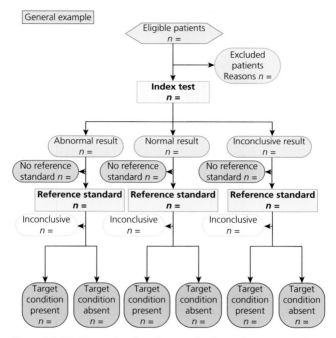

Figure 5.2 STARD's template flow diagram of a diagnostic accuracy study. (Reproduced from www.stard-statement.org with permission from STARD.)

CHAPTER 6
Sources of bias in diagnostic studies

Bias is important to consider when appraising a study. A biased study may produce a result that is 'wrong'. However, biases are often unavoidable even in well-conducted diagnostic studies. This does not mean that you should discard the study, but rather that you should consider what effects they might have on the results of the study.

There are many possible sources of bias to be aware of in diagnostic studies.

WHAT ARE THE KEY BIASES?
1. Spectrum bias (or selection bias)
2. Verification bias (or referral or work-up bias)
3. Incorporation bias
4. Observer bias (or test review bias)
5. Differential reference bias (or double gold standard bias)

Spectrum bias (also known as selection bias)
A study may select patients who are healthier, or more unwell, than patients whom we would see in real life. In such circumstances, there would be bias in the results. Ideally the spectrum of patients (or study participants) used in the diagnostic study should be similar to the types of patients for whom the test is intended. Spectrum or selection bias occurs when study participants have been chosen who are not representative of the real-life clinical situation.

Selecting a more severe spectrum of patients who have the disease will tend to inflate sensitivity. A healthier spectrum of patients in the non-diseased group will tend to increase the specificity.

The following example illustrates this: the clock-drawing test is used to assess cognitive function. Clearly, people residing in nursing homes with advanced dementia would experience difficulties in performing the test, i.e. most would test 'positive', thus leading to near-perfect sensitivity. Alternatively, college students would probably have little difficulty in performing the test, i.e. most would test 'negative', thus leading to near-perfect specificity.

Diagnostic Tests Toolkit, First Edition. Matthew Thompson, Ann Van den Bruel.
© 2012 John Wiley & Sons, Ltd. Published 2012 by John Wiley & Sons, Ltd.

The ideal way of selecting patients for a diagnostic study is by using consecutive recruitment of patients.

Figure 6.1 illustrates how selective inclusion might distort the results. From the entire population, only a proportion are selected and get the index and reference standard. The subjects who were not selected for the study might well differ in terms of disease severity, prognosis, response to treatment, etc.

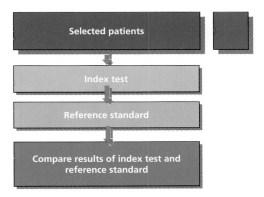

Figure 6.1

For example, let's say that you want to determine the accuracy of an exercise ECG test (index test) for diagnosing angina, compared with coronary angiography (reference standard) in the accident and emergency department. All patients in whom angina might reasonably be suspected go on to have the index test and reference standard. *Spectrum bias* occurs when the study selects only those patients in whom you are almost certain that they have angina, e.g. those who are already scheduled to undergo angiography and subsequent percutaneous intervention.

SPECTRUM BIAS: CAN IT BE AVOIDED?
This type of selection is common in many diagnostic studies, because it is often impossible to perform a diagnostic test that may have some costs or harms associated with it (e.g. potential exposure to X-rays, costs of the test) in all patients who might possibly have the target condition. It is often necessary to make a pragmatic clinical judgement about the degree of selection used in the study, and whether it is reasonable or not.

Verification bias (also called referral or work-up bias)

Ideally all patients in the diagnostic study have an index test performed and then have the reference test. Verification bias occurs when only some of the patients who have the index test go on to have the reference standard. Typically this means that patients who are positive on the index test are the ones who go on to have the reference standard, whereas those who have a negative index test don't get the reference standard performed.

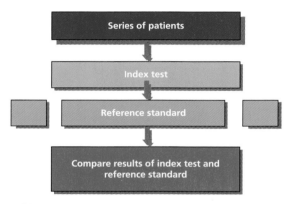

Figure 6.2

For example, returning to our study comparing how accurately an exercise ECG ('treadmill test') identifies patients with angina compared with coronary angiography. *Ideally* all patients who get a treadmill ECG test then go on to get coronary angiography. *Verification bias* occurs when only those patients who have a positive exercise ECG test go on to have angiography performed.

VERIFICATION BIAS: CAN IT BE AVOIDED?
It may be difficult to perform a reference test in all patients,
particularly if it is more invasive or risky (as in the case of
coronary angiography).

Alternative options might include following up patients who test negative
with the index test over time to see if they develop the target condition. If
the target condition is rapidly progressive or even fatal without treatment,
then it is reasonable to assume that the reference test is negative if the
patient did not experience this unfavourable outcome. Verification bias is
more problematic for conditions that have a subclinical or self-limiting
course; they will be more easily missed if the reference standard is not
performed on everyone.

Incorporation bias

The index test should be compared with an independent reference
standard. However, sometimes the reference standard actually includes
(or incorporates) part of the index test being evaluated. In other words the
reference standard is defined in part by a positive index test. This will tend
to make an index test perform very accurately.

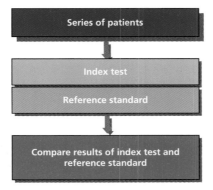

Figure 6.3

For example, we are interested in assessing how well a new inflammatory
marker performs for diagnosing exacerbations of inflammatory arthritis.
However, the definition of exacerbations of arthritis is based on a
combination of symptoms (e.g. worse joint pain, fatigue) as well as raised
levels of inflammatory markers.

Ideally it would be better to have a reference standard for this disease that does not include the index test. *Incorporation bias* occurs when the definition of exacerbations of inflammatory arthritis is based partly on the presence of a positive inflammatory blood test.

INCORPORATION BIAS: CAN IT BE AVOIDED?
In many clinical conditions, the reference standard does include many features, rather than a single test, so it may not be possible to avoid. If there is incorporation bias and the index test does not perform well, then this information is likely to be true. Also, where there is incorporation bias the diagnostic study may be answering a slightly different question – not 'How well does the index test diagnose the target condition?' but rather 'How well does the index text predict the diagnosis of the target condition?' (i.e. clinician performance).

Observer (or test review bias) bias

Ideally the results of the index test should be compared with the results of the reference standard by an observer who is blinded, i.e. who is not aware of the results of the index test. Bias can occur when the individual who is performing (or interpreting) the reference standard knows the results of the index test. This can potentially lead to bias because he or she may perform or interpret the reference test differently, depending on the results of the index test (and vice versa). This is particularly a problem for tests whose interpretation is more subjective. It can also be a problem for tests where the researcher is able to choose the threshold or cut-off between positive and negative (or normal and abnormal) in order to maximize one component of diagnostic accuracy.

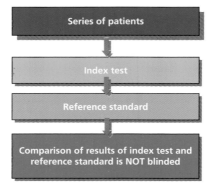

Figure 6.4

For example, returning to our example of determining the accuracy of exercise ECG for identifying patients with angina, compared with a reference standard of coronary angiography. In this case let's assume that everyone has both the index test and the reference standard performed.

Ideally the results of the index test and reference standard are compared with each other by a member of the research team who is not aware of the results of each of them. *Observer bias* occurs when the researcher who is interpreting the results of the angiography knows what the exercise ECG showed (i.e. he or she is not blinded), so perhaps might look more closely at the results of the angiography in patients with positive exercise ECGs.

OBSERVER BIAS: CAN IT BE AVOIDED?
In a research setting it should be possible to keep the comparison of the results of the index test and reference standard blinded.

However, in some clinical studies it may be difficult to entirely separate these.

Differential reference bias (double gold standard)

This occurs when some of the patients in a study have one reference standard, and others have a different reference standard applied, depending on the results of the index test. This might happen in situations where the reference standard is invasive, so it would be only likely (or ethical) to perform it in patients who have a positive result on their index test. For some clinical conditions there is no accepted reference standard; these are often the conditions where new tests are being evaluated.

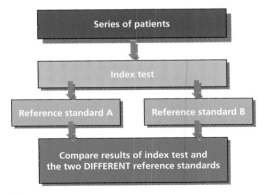

Figure 6.5

For example, let's say that you want to compare how well the treadmill test identifies patients with angina compared with coronary angiography. *Ideally* all patients get angiography as the reference standard, regardless of whether their ECG treadmill test was positive or negative.

Differential reference bias occurs when patients who have a positive (or perhaps equivocal) exercise ECG test go on to have angiography performed, whereas those who have a negative ECG test just get followed up as outpatients over time to see if they clinically develop angina.

DIFFERENTIAL REFERENCE BIAS: CAN IT BE AVOIDED?

It is difficult to apply the same reference standard to all patients in a study, particularly if a reference test is more invasive or costly, or has potential side effects (as in the case of coronary angiography or biopsies). In these cases it may be possible to use a combination of several less invasive reference tests, or use follow-up over time.

What are the effects of the different design-related biases?

Identifying the biases in a diagnostic study is important in order to determine how the biases might affect the results of the study and the conclusions that you draw from it.

TIP

Studies performed using the *same* test can give *different* values for diagnostic accuracy, depending on the study design.

However, many diagnostic studies will have potential biases, and it would be wrong to discard them without considering what effects (if any) these are likely to have on the results. Based on two large systematic reviews of published papers (Lijmer et al. 1999; Rutjes et al. 2006), some design features seem to have a greater impact on the accuracy estimates in diagnostic studies than other features.

The way that patients are selected seems to be the most important source of bias. Several design features can lead to diagnostic accuracy being *overestimated*:

- Non-consecutive recruitment of patients.
- Case–control studies, where cases with severe illness are selected, and controls are healthy individuals. Indeed, case–control studies might

overestimate the diagnostic odds ratio (DOR) by almost fivefold, compared with studies that recruited patients using a cohort.
- Data collected retrospectively or routinely collected clinical data.
- Differential verification, i.e. studies that used two or more different reference tests to verify the results of the index test

In contrast, the only study design feature that was associated with significant *underestimation* of diagnostic accuracy was when patients were selected based on whether they had been referred for the index test, compared with studies that included all patients with some prespecified symptoms or signs of the target condition.

Further reading

Jaeschke R, Guyatt G, Sackett DL. Users' guides to the medical literature. III. How to use an article about a diagnostic test. A. Are the results of the study valid? Evidence-Based Medicine Working Group. *JAMA* 1994;**271**:389–91.

Knottnerus JA, Leffers P. The influence of referral patterns on the characteristics of diagnostic tests. *J Clin Epidemiol* 1992;**45**:1143–54.

Lijmer JG, Mol BW, Heisterkamp S, et al. Empirical evidence of design-related bias in studies of diagnostic tests. *JAMA* 1999;**282**:1061–6

Montori VM, Wyer P, Newman TB, et al. Tips for learners of evidence-based medicine: 5. The effect of spectrum of disease on the performance of diagnostic tests. *Can Med Assoc J* 2005;**173**:385–90.

Rutjes AW, Reitsma JB, Di Nisio M, et al. Evidence of bias and variation in diagnostic accuracy studies. *Can Med Assoc J* 2006;**174**;469–76

Glas AS, Bossuyt PM, Kleijnen J. Sources of variation and bias in studies of diagnostic accuracy. *Ann Intern Med* 2004;**140**:189–202.

CHAPTER 7
Measures of discrimination of diagnostic tests

Two by two tables

The results of diagnostic accuracy studies are commonly summarized in two by two (2 × 2) tables.

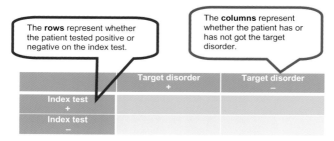

The **rows** represent whether the patient tested positive or negative on the index test.

The **columns** represent whether the patient has or has not got the target disorder.

	Target disorder +	Target disorder −
Index test +		
Index test −		

Figure 7.1

Do not alter the direction of the table. ⚠

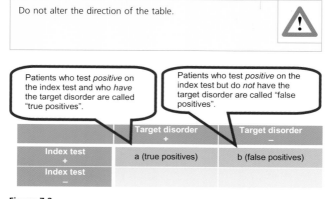

Patients who test *positive* on the index test and who *have* the target disorder are called "true positives".

Patients who test *positive* on the index test but do *not* have the target disorder are called "false positives".

	Target disorder +	Target disorder −
Index test +	a (true positives)	b (false positives)
Index test −		

Figure 7.2

Diagnostic Tests Toolkit, First Edition. Matthew Thompson, Ann Van den Bruel.
© 2012 John Wiley & Sons, Ltd. Published 2012 by John Wiley & Sons, Ltd.

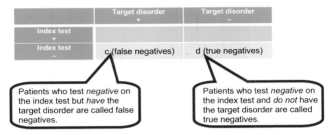

	Target disorder +	Target disorder −
Index test +		
Index test −	c (false negatives)	d (true negatives)

Patients who test *negative* on the index test but *have* the target disorder are called false negatives.

Patients who test *negative* on the index test and *do not* have the target disorder are called true negatives.

Figure 7.3

Example: we are interested in looking at the accuracy of exercise ECG tests (the *index test*) in the diagnosis of coronary artery disease (the *target disorder*). We have 90 patients who had a positive exercise test and who we know have coronary artery disease (true positives):

	Target disorder +	Target disorder −
Index test +	90	b (false positives)
Index test −	c (false negatives)	d (true negatives)

But there are 50 people who had a positive exercise test who did not in fact have any coronary artery disease (false positives).

	Target disorder +	Target disorder −
Index test +	90	50
Index test −	c (false negatives)	d (true negatives)

Another 50 people had a negative exercise test and did not have coronary artery disease (true negatives).

	Target disorder +	Target disorder −
Index test +	90	50
Index test −	c (false negatives)	50

Finally, 10 people had a negative exercise test although they did in fact have coronary artery disease (false negatives).

	Target disorder +	Target disorder −
Index test +	90	50
Index test −	10	50

Outcome measures

The value of the index test can be expressed in various measures derived from a single 2 × 2 table.

Sensitivity is the probability of a positive (abnormal) test result in individuals with the target disorder:

$$Sens = \frac{a}{a+c}$$

In our example, sensitivity = 90/(90 + 10) = 90/100 = 0.9 (mostly expressed as 90%):

	Target disorder +	Target disorder −
Index test +	90 (a)	
Index test −	10 (c)	

Specificity is the probability of a negative (normal) test result in participants without the target disorder.

$$Spec = \frac{d}{b+d}$$

In our example, specificity = 50 / (50 + 50) = 50 / 100 = 0.5 (or 50%)

	Target disorder +	Target disorder −
Index test +		50 (b)
Index test −		50 (d)

Positive predictive value (PPV) is the probability of the target disorder in participants with a positive (abnormal) test result.

$$PPV = \frac{a}{a+b}$$

In our example, the PPV = 90 / (90 + 50) = 90 / 140 = 0.6 (or 64%).

	Target disorder +	Target disorder −
Index test +	90 (a)	50 (b)
Index test −		

Negative predictive value (NPV) is the probability of absence of the target disorder in participants with a negative (normal) test result.

$$NPV = \frac{d}{c+d}$$

In our example, the NPV = 50 / (50 + 10) = 0.83 (or 83%).

	Target disorder +	Target disorder −
Index test +		
Index test −	10 (c)	50 (d)

Positive likelihood ratio (LR+) shows how many times more likely patients with the target disorder are to have a positive test result than patients without the target disorder.

$$LR+ = \frac{Sens}{1-Spec} = \frac{\dfrac{a}{a+c}}{\dfrac{b}{b+d}}$$

In our example, the LR+ = 1.8.

	Target disorder +	Target disorder −
Index test +	90 (a)	50 (b)
Index test −	10 (c)	50 (d)

The **negative likelihood ratio** (LR−) shows how many times less likely patients with the target disorder are to have a negative test result than patients without the target disorder.

$$LR- = \frac{1 - Sens}{Spec} = \frac{\frac{c}{a+c}}{\frac{d}{b+d}}$$

In our example, the LR− = 0.2.

The **diagnostic odds ratio** (DOR) is a single value that represents the overall discrimination of a test.

$$OR = \frac{ad}{bc}$$

In our example, the OR = 9.

The **prevalence** of the target disorder in the sample is the number of patients with the target condition in the entire sample.

Prevalence is also referred to as the pre-test probability: the probability of having the target disorder before performing the index test.

$$Prevalence = \frac{a+c}{a+b+c+d}$$

In our example, the prevalence = 100/200 = 50%.

	Target disorder +	Target disorder −
Index test +	90 (a)	50 (b)
Index test −	10 (c)	50 (d)
	100 (a + c)	100 (b + d)

Which measure should you use and why?

All of these measures tell you something slightly different about the test. Sensitivity and specificity tell you how many of the subjects *with or without the target disorder* a test can identify. Predictive values and likelihood ratios tell you something about how much more likely the target disorder is, *given a certain test result*.

> SpPin
> SnNout

Some people use the SpPin–SnNout rule of thumb, meaning that high specificity allows ruling in and high sensitivity allows ruling out. This is because, when sensitivity is high, there are few false negatives, so that it would be unusual for patients to have the target condition but have a negative index test. And when specificity is high, there are few false positives, so it would be unusual for patients without the target condition to have a positive index test.

In clinical practice, predictive values and likelihood ratios are more useful, because generally you don't know if the patient does or does not have the condition (that is probably why you are doing the test in the first place!). Predictive values and likelihood ratios reason from the results of the index test and not from the disease status of the patient.

> Predictive values are directly dependent on the prevalence, more about this later.

The diagnostic odds ratio offers a single overall measure of discrimination, allowing comparison across tests. However, most tests are asymmetrical, i.e. better at ruling in a target disorder than at ruling out, or vice versa. This asymmetry is concealed in the odds ratio, which makes it less informative for clinical practice.

Let's go back to the example we used earlier. The sensitivity of the test was 90% and the specificity 50%. The odds ratio is 9.

	Target disorder +	Target disorder −
Index test +	90 (*a*)	50 (*b*)
Index test −	10 (*c*)	50 (*d*)

Sensitivity $a/(a + c)$: 90%
Specificity $d/(b + d)$: 50%
LR+ sens/(1 − spec): 1.8
LR− (1 − sens)/spec: 0.2
OR: ad/bc: 9
PPV: $a/(a + b)$: 64.3%
NPV: $d/(c + d)$: 83.3%

Now let us look at a different index test, which has opposite sensitivity and specificity (50% and 90% respectively). This time when we calculate the odds ratio, it is again 9.

Different sensitivity and specificity, but *identical* odds ratio.

	Target disorder +	Target disorder −
Index test +	50 (*a*)	10 (*b*)
Index test −	50 (*c*)	90 (*d*)

Sensitivity *a*/(*a* + *c*): 50%
Specificity *d*/(*b* + *d*): 90%
LR+ sens/(1 − spec): 5.0
LR− (1 − sens)/spec: 0.5
OR: *ad*/*bc*: 9
PPV: *a*/(*a* + *b*): 83.3%
NPV: *d*/(*c* + *d*): 64.3%

Note that *both* index tests have odds ratios of 9, despite having very different sensitivity and specificity and the same prevalence of 50%.

In the first table, patients testing positive will have a 64% chance of having the target disorder if the index test is positive (PPV), and a 17% chance if the index test is negative (1 − NPV). This index test is therefore better at *ruling out* the target disorder than at ruling it in, because the change from 50% to 17% is more important than the change from 50% to 64%.

In the second table, patients testing positive on the index test will have a chance of 83% of having the target disorder (PPV) and patients testing negative will have a chance of 36% of having the target disorder. This shows that this test is good at *ruling in* the target disorder rather than ruling it out: there is a more meaningful change in probability from 50% to 83% than from 50% to 36%.

So, tests with identical odds ratios can be totally different in their ability to rule in or rule out the target disorder.

The effect of prevalence on predictive values

As we have already hinted, predictive values are directly dependent on prevalence. What this means is that the same test will have a different predictive value in a different population. This seriously limits the usefulness of positive and negative predictive values.

Below is an example of an index test with identical sensitivity, specificity, and thus identical likelihood ratios and odds ratio to our initial example.

The only difference is the prevalence of the target condition. In the earlier example, prevalence was 50%; here prevalence is lower at 33%. Comparing these two tables, it is clear that predictive values will change as the prevalence changes.

In the first table (prevalence of 50%), the sensitivity was 90% and specificity 50%, the PPV was 83% and the NPV 64%.

But now, when the prevalence is lower (33%), and with the same sensitivity and specificity, the PPV is now 47% and the NPV 91% – lower prevalence with identical sensitivity and specificity.

	Target disorder +	Target disorder −
Index test +	90 (a)	100 (b)
Index test −	10 (c)	100 (d)

Sensitivity $a/(a + c)$: 90%
Specificity $d/(b + d)$: 50%
LR+ sens/(1 − spec): 1.8
LR− (1 − sens)/spec: 0.2
OR: ad/bc: 9
PPV: $a/(a + b)$: 47.4%
NPV: $d/(c + d)$: 90.9%

Based on this theoretical example, sensitivity and specificity, and as a consequence likelihood ratios, appear to be unaffected by changes in prevalence. However, studies have found that these measures of diagnostic accuracy do indeed vary across populations with different prevalences. This is because prevalence in itself is a proxy for other changes that influence the diagnostic value of tests. In general, this can be caused by changes in those having the target condition or by changes in those not having the target condition. For example, fever exceeding 40°C has good diagnostic value for serious infections in children in primary care where prevalence is low, but not in secondary care where prevalence is higher. This is explained by the fact that children presenting to secondary care have been selected, among other things based on temperature. In other words, on average, many more children in secondary care will have high fever, limiting the usefulness of fever in that setting. More on this later.

Effect of time on diagnostic accuracy

As illnesses are usually dynamic processes, time can affect diagnostic accuracy between settings with different prevalences. Typically you would expect patients in primary care to have shorter and therefore less advanced stages of many illnesses than patients in secondary care. It is usually fair to assume that it is easier to detect a target condition in a more advanced stage, because more of the pathophysiological changes that your test is aimed at will have had time to occur by then.

Infectious diseases are typical examples of the influence of time on diagnostic process. For example, infection with *Neisseria meningitidis* causes meningococcal meningitis and sepsis. The classic features of this disease, namely haemorrhagic rash, neck stiffness and impaired consciousness, only develop 13–22 h after the start of the illness. Before this time only general signs of illness such as fever are present. Thus in the early stages of this disease, the (absence of) neck stiffness provides little diagnostic value, yet only hours later it will be extremely useful for diagnosis.

Effect of severity of the target condition on diagnostic accuracy

A similar but not identical mechanism is the severity of the target condition. Patients with a 'mild case' of the target condition may not exhibit the feature at which the index test is aimed. For example, patients with a mild degree of heart failure may not have shortness of breath on exertion.

The referral filter

Another mechanism introducing changes in spectrum is prior testing and subsequent referral from one level of care to another. This process selects patients based on presenting features, related to the target condition or to other conditions mimicking the target condition. This leads to a selection of patients with a higher probability of the target condition but also with co-morbidities that are difficult to distinguish from the target condition.

For example, consider patients who are referred to a hospital surgical unit with suspicion of appendicitis: many will present with pain in the right lower quadrant of the abdomen, because this sign is used by primary care physicians to refer patients to secondary care. Consequently, pain in the right lower quadrant will *no longer discriminate* between patients with and those without appendicitis in the hospital surgical unit setting.

Thus, all outcome measures can be affected by changes in the setting and prevalence. It is a safe assumption that diagnostic accuracy differs across settings unless proven otherwise.

Bayesian reasoning

Likelihood ratios are very useful for clinical practice, because they allow calculation of the change in probability of the target condition, for patients with a positive or a negative index test.

This is done using Bayes' theorem. Bayesian mathematics enables us to re-calculate the probability of the disease once the result from a given test is known. In other words, Bayes' theorem shows that the probability of the target disorder given a positive or negative index test (post-test probability) depends on the pre-test probability and the diagnostic accuracy of the index test.

Mathematically, Bayes' theorem is calculated as shown in the box.

Pretest probability = p1
Pretest odds = o1 = p1/(1 − p1)
Post-test odds = o2 = pretest odds × likelihood ratio = o1 × LR
Post-test probability = p2 = o2/(1 + o2)

An easy way to avoid these calculations is to use Fagan's nomogram, which shows the change in probability after applying the index test. This is most useful for reporting the results of a single index test. In studies where multiple results are reported, either because there is more than one index test or more than one population/subgroups, these nomograms are less useful.

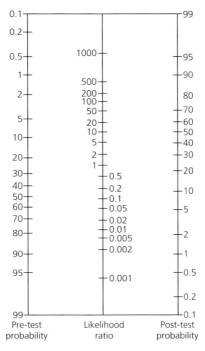

Figure 7.4 Fagan's nomogram.

Starting from the pre-test probability on the left axis, and using the likelihood ratios, the nomogram shows the post-test probability for a positive and negative test result respectively.

For example, let us say the pre-test probability for a patient with chest pain presenting to accident and emergency for myocardial infarction is 5% (Figure 7.5). If the patient is sweating (LR+ 2.06), the post-test probability increases to 10% (green arrow). If the patient is not sweating (LR– 0.65), the post-test probability of a myocardial infarction lowers slightly to 3% (red arrow).

Rules of thumb for interpreting likelihood ratios

The following rules of thumb are a useful way of categorizing how useful a likelihood ratio is expected to be:

- LRs >10 or <0.1 generate large, and often conclusive, changes from pre- to post-test probability.
- LRs of 5–10 and 0.1–0.2 generate moderate shifts in probability.
- LRs of 2–5 and 0.5–0.2 generate small (but sometimes important) changes in probability.
- LRs of 1–2 and 0.5–1 alter probability to a very small and rarely important degree.

The earlier example of sweating in patients with chest pain is an example of a test that only moderately changes the probability of a myocardial infarction after either a positive or a negative test. Again, tests can have an asymmetrical value, e.g. a positive test might generate large changes in probability whereas a negative test only small changes.

A resting ECG showing ST-segment elevation has a higher positive LR (13) and a similar negative LR (0.47) than sweating for the diagnosis of myocardial infarction. Assuming that the pre-test probability is the same, the presence of ST elevation changes the probability of myocardial infarction to 41%, whereas the absence of ST elevation changes the probability to 2% (Figure 7.6).

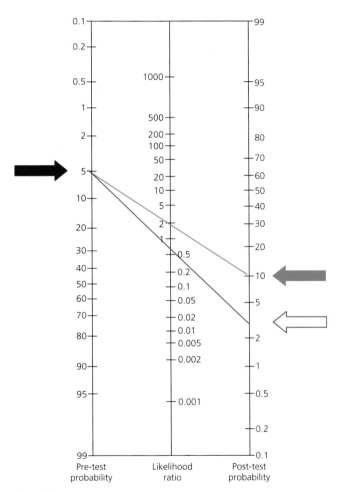

Figure 7.5

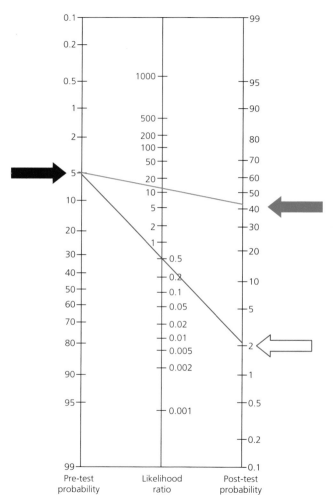

Figure 7.6

> Changes in probability are most important when prevalence is moderately high, around 40–80%.
>
> In low prevalence and high prevalence, changes in probability are smaller.

Tests that have more than two result categories

Until now, we have focused on tests that have only two possible results, either positive or negative. However, many tests used in clinical practice have more than two outcomes. Some tests have multiple possible results or categories (such as the CAGE questionnaire for screening for alcohol abuse) and others may be continuous (e.g. many laboratory tests).

What should you do when you cannot seem to summarize the results into a simple 2 × 2 table? In many cases results are dichotomized, i.e. forced into two categories, so that the results can be fitted into a 2 × 2 table. However, this causes a great loss of information, comparable to throwing away a third of the data. Obviously that reduces your statistical power! In addition, any non-linear relationship between the index test and the target condition is concealed.

If, nevertheless, the data are dichotomized, then the cut-point used should be chosen in advance rather than choosing an optimal cut-point depending on the results.

For tests with more than two categories, likelihood ratios can be computed for each category. The likelihood ratio for that category then represents the ratio of the probability of a given outcome category among diseased and the probability of that given outcome category among non-diseased individuals. For example, the results for CAGE questionnaire on alcohol misuse are categorized as negative (zero 'yes' answers), 1–2 'yes' answers and 3–4 'yes' answers. The likelihood ratio for 3–4 'yes' answers is the ratio of the probability of having 3–4 'yes' answers in people *with* an alcohol problem over the probability of having 3–4 'yes' answers in people *without* an alcohol problem.

	Target disorder +	Target disorder −
Index test +	a	b
Index test intermediate	e	f
Index test −	c	d

Likelihood ratio of a positive test result:

$$LR+ = \dfrac{\dfrac{a}{a+e+c}}{\dfrac{b}{b+f+d}}$$

Likelihood ratio of an intermediate test result:

$$LR\ intermediate = \dfrac{\dfrac{e}{a+e+c}}{\dfrac{f}{b+f+d}}$$

Likelihood ratio of a negative test result:

$$LR- = \dfrac{\dfrac{c}{a+e+c}}{\dfrac{d}{b+f+d}}$$

If an index test has an intermediate level, it is important that this level is analysed separately and not simply 'lumped together' with the positive or negative test results, or omitted from the analyses altogether (as sometimes happens!). If the intermediate level is wrongly included in either the positive or the negative results, this leads to inaccurate estimates of sensitivity and specificity. If it is included with the positive results it will underestimate sensitivity and overestimate specificity, whereas if it is included with the negative results it will overestimate sensitivity and underestimate specificity.

ROC curves

The results of tests with multiple categories or truly continuous tests may be summarized in receiver operating characteristic (ROC) curves. The purpose of these graphs is to explore the performance of the test where different levels are used as the 'cut-off' to define a positive or negative test result. For example, breathing rate in normal infants varies between 40 and 60 breaths/min. Breathing rate is considered too fast (possibly caused by pneumonia) when it is 60 breaths/min or higher. This value (≥60 breaths/min) is thus used as a *cut-off* to define abnormal breathing rates. But, it is possible to use different cut-offs, say 65 or 70 breaths/min, to define an abnormal breathing rate. At each cut-off, the sensitivity and 1 − specificity (false positive rate) of breathing rate compared with the reference standard for pneumonia (such as a chest radiograph) are plotted in ROC space.

ROC space is defined by the true positive rate (i.e. sensitivity) on the y axis, and the false-positive rate (i.e. 1 − specificity) on the x axis. Both axes go from 0 to 100%, although they are sometimes labelled as 0–1.0. Sometimes you will see the x axis labelled as specificity (not 1 − specificity) with values from 100% at the origin to 0% at the right hand end – this is just another way of saying the same thing.

For example, a test with 30% sensitivity and 90% specificity (10% false-positive rate) is plotted in the lower left corner (Figure 7.7).

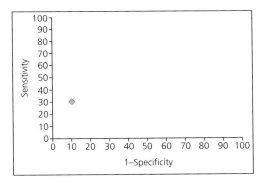

Figure 7.7

If that test has another cut-point with a sensitivity of 60% and a specificity of 80%, the second point is plotted, as in Figure 7.8.

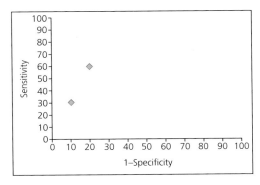

Figure 7.8

Continuing with other cut-points (Figure 7.9).

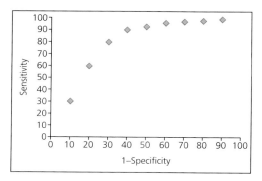

Figure 7.9

A test that does *not provide any* diagnostic information would be plotted on the diagonal as shown below. All the points on the diagonal have sensitivity = 1 − specificity. So, at a sensitivity of 20% the 1 − specificity would be 20%, and at a sensitivity of 40% the 1 − specificity would be 40%, and so on. At all these points, the likelihood ratios are equal to 1, providing no change in the probability of the target condition (Figure 7.10).

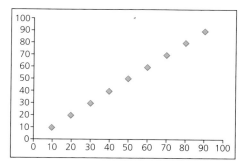

Figure 7.10

In contrast, a *perfect* test result (100% sensitivity and 100% specificity) lies in the upper left corner. ROC curves that approach that left upper corner have better diagnostic accuracy than tests with a curve approaching the diagonal (Figure 7.11).

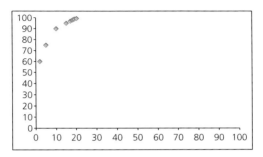

Figure 7.11

The area under the curve (AUC) is an overall measure of test performance that allows comparison between tests. The AUC ranges from 0.5 for a useless test (i.e. the curve lying on the diagonal) to 1.0 for a perfect test.

The shape of the ROC curve allows the identification of a range or cut-off that best suits clinical practice. For example, where a test is used for triage of a potential life-threatening illness, sensitivity would need to be maximized whereas moderate specificity may be acceptable.

In the example of white blood cell count in Figure 7.12, sensitivity is very high at a cut-off point of ≥10 000 cells/mm³, corresponding to a sensitivity of 93% and a specificity of 43% (green arrow). If, on the other hand, the clinical goal of the test is to rule in a target disorder before starting treatment let us say, then specificity would be more important and a cut-off of ≥20 000 cells/mm³, which provides a sensitivity of 38% and specificity of 92% would be more appropriate (red arrow).

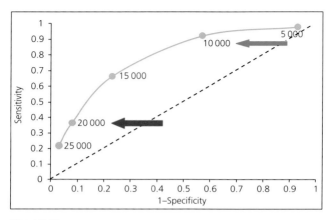

Figure 7.12

Further reading

Altman DG. Problems in dichotomizing continuous variables. *Am J Epidemiol* 1994;**139**:442–5.

Deeks JJ, Altman DG. Sensitivity and specificity and their confidence intervals cannot exceed 100%. *BMJ* 1999;**318**:193–4.

Jaeschke R, Guyatt GH, Sackett DL. Users' guides to the medical literature. III. How to use an article about a diagnostic test. B. What are the results and will they help me in caring for my patients? The Evidence-Based Medicine Working Group. *JAMA* 1994;**271**:703–7.

Leeflang MM, Bossuyt PM, Irwig L. Diagnostic test accuracy may vary with prevalence: implications for evidence-based diagnosis. *J Clin Epidemiol* 2009;**62**:5–12.

Perera R, Heneghan C. Making sense of diagnostic test likelihood ratios. *ACP J Club* 2007;**146**:A8–9.

CHAPTER 8
Using diagnostic information in clinical practice

In clinical practice, diagnosis involves more than simply applying the results from a single 2 × 2 table. In general, clinicians collect several different types of information about a patient, and combine this information in multiple ways to make diagnoses. Evidence-based diagnosis aims to highlight the most efficient use of tests.

Diagnostic information from patients includes presenting symptoms, responses to questions about the presence or absence of symptoms, and examination findings. This is complemented by further tests, some of which may be simple point-of-care diagnostic tests (e.g. urine analysis, ECG), whereas others include imaging and laboratory tests involving clinical pathology, biochemistry, haematology, etc. Moreover, these components of diagnostic information may be collected at one consultation, or as a series of tests *over time* during several consultations.

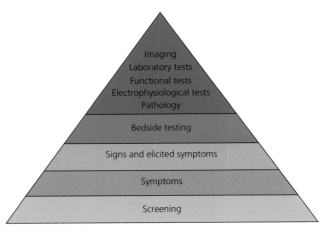

Figure 8.1

Diagnostic Tests Toolkit, First Edition. Matthew Thompson, Ann Van den Bruel.
© 2012 John Wiley & Sons, Ltd. Published 2012 by John Wiley & Sons, Ltd.

Validity of data

With all types of clinical information, it is worth asking how valid the information is, i.e. how closely does the information represent the actual or true situation?

WHAT ARE THE THREE KEY ASPECTS TO VALIDITY?
1. Face validity
2. Predictive validity
3. Concurrent validity

---

1. Face validity: is the test a reasonable tool for this condition? For example, an ankle radiograph is a reasonable way to diagnose ankle injuries, but not to assess the presence of tonsillitis (obviously!).
2. Predictive validity: how well does the test predict the final diagnosis? These are the measures of diagnostic accuracy discussed in Chapter 7.
3. Concurrent validity: how well do two different forms of information agree? For example, does a patient's subjective complaint of having difficulty breathing agree with an objective measure of respiratory function?

THE BALANCE BETWEEN OVER-DIAGNOSIS AND UNDER-DIAGNOSIS
The level of diagnostic uncertainty that an individual clinician is prepared to accept depends on personal characteristics, type of clinical practice and health-care setting.

Some clinicians are more confident in their diagnostic skills than others, whereas some can be inappropriately confident (i.e. they lack sufficient experience). Primary care or generalist specialties tacitly involve greater acceptance of uncertainty as a broad spectrum of patients present with a wide variety of clinical conditions, at different time points in their illnesses. In these settings accepting a certain level of diagnostic uncertainty is important.

In other clinical settings the acceptability of uncertainty will be far lower – these include clinical specialties that focus on more narrow disease areas, referred patients (e.g. secondary or tertiary care) or where therapeutic decisions are even more critical. Understanding these varying thresholds for uncertainty is important, and it is equally important to communicate diagnostic uncertainty with patients. Acceptance of appropriate risk is also fundamental to the functioning of a health-care system, and concerns about medical malpractice, for example, can often result in higher use of diagnostic testing.

UNDER-TESTING
Failure to use sufficient (or correct) tests to identify the true disease stated in appropriate time.

OVER-TESTING
Tests are applied inefficiently or excessively. Can lead to inappropriate (and potentially costly) additional tests, referral or treatment.

Problem-solving strategies that clinicians use in diagnosis

Psychologists have tried to explain some of the diagnostic decision-making (reasoning) processes that clinicians use when solving clinical diagnostic problems. This has led to several theories.

Hypothetical deductive reasoning

Clinicians collect information on a selected limited number of possible diagnoses (hypotheses) and rank them. Further clinical information that is collected is then used to add or remove hypotheses and re-rank them in a repeating process. This suggests that clinicians make a relatively small number of diagnostic hypotheses early on in the consultation, and these are what guide the further gathering of information from clinical examination for example. Experienced clinicians may start with fewer and more accurate hypotheses than novices.

Categorization

The way that we apply (or generalize) knowledge about a limited set of objects, and apply it to new previously unseen objects, is a key concept in human intelligence (i.e. our brains are not surprised every time we see a new car because we use knowledge from previous cars to interpret it). In clinical reasoning, this might occur in different ways. One theory suggests that clinicians 'average' experiences with individual cases into a prototype case, so when a new case is experienced it can be compared feature by feature to see what it has in common. This might be helpful for novice clinicians in particular. An alternative theory states that, rather than this feature-by-feature comparison, in fact what may happen is that over time a large number of instances or exemplars are collected, and when a new case is encountered it is mentally matched against an exemplar or instance (how does it compare to instances of this seen before?), or indeed against a hypothetical case (what the case is supposed to present with).

In reality, clinicians use several different methods of reasoning, often within the same consultation. An illustration of this process comes from a study of experienced family doctors in Oxford, who recorded the diagnostic strategies that they used when making diagnoses in their patients in primary care clinics. Using this information the researchers proposed a three-stage model of diagnostic reasoning: initiation of diagnostic hypotheses, refinement of these diagnostic hypotheses and definition of the final diagnosis. Within each of these stages, clinicians used various diagnostic strategies.

Stages and strategies in arriving at a diagnosis

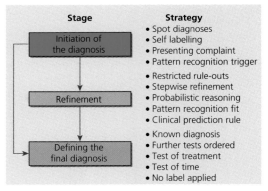

Heneghan C et al. BMJ 2009;338:bmj.b946
©2009 by British Medical Journal Publishing Group

Figure 8.2 Stages and strategies in arriving at a diagnosis.

WHAT CAN GO WRONG?
Applying these diagnostic problem-solving strategies is not straightforward, and clinicians can develop various biases or heuristics (i.e. rules of thumb) which may impede their diagnostic decision-making.

For example:
- Failure to even generate or consider a relevant hypothesis.
- Representativeness: assumes that a patient who has one feature in common with a group of patients with a given target condition must have that condition.
- Cue blindness: ignoring clinical information that does not seem to 'fit'.
- Confirmatory bias: stops looking for more diagnostic information too early in the consultation.
- Availability: the relative ease with which some events are remembered (e.g. memorable cases, missed diagnoses) affects how probable a diagnosis is. Over-estimates the frequency with which rare or unusual cases will occur (perhaps ones that receive a lot of media attention), and under-estimates the frequency of cases that are less exciting or memorable.
- Anchoring: the tendency to latch onto the first diagnosis that springs to mind, and not change.

Action thresholds versus testing thresholds ('Will the test change my management?')

Patients who obviously have a condition may not need any further tests to confirm the diagnosis (or may need only some of the tests, e.g. to assess its severity) – in other words they have reached a threshold for action. For example, a patient presenting to a family doctor with crushing central chest pain and sweating who has a past history of ischaemic heart disease has crossed the action threshold, and needs something done (in this case immediate referral for hospital treatment for possible unstable angina or myocardial infarction [MI]). Additional tests in the clinic (such as an ECG) at this point may simply waste time – the diagnostic threshold for doing something has clearly been passed. This is related to the important concept that diagnosis itself does not usually affect patient outcomes; it is the *actions* that the clinician or patient take subsequently that alter outcomes.

At the other end of the probability spectrum is the patient who obviously does not have the condition of interest, so that it is 'not worth' doing a test. For example, a fit young man presenting with a slight chest wall pain that seems worse on moving his arm is highly unlikely to have ischaemic heart disease, and more likely to have a muscle strain. Most clinicians would examine for other causes of his symptoms and perhaps other testing; however, he almost certainly does not need an ECG – in other words he has not reached the threshold where it is worth testing.

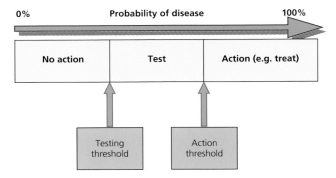

Figure 8.3

Methods for combining test results

Diagnosis in clinical practice is seldom based on the results of a single test. In reality, clinicians use combinations of baseline information about a patient (e.g. age and gender), clinical features and various additional tests. There are several possible methods for analysing the diagnostic value of multiple tests, some of which can include more than one target disorder. However, the diagnostic value of two tests is not independent. In other words, the diagnostic value of test A changes when test B is also used. There are several possible techniques for analysing the diagnostic value of multiple tests, some of which can include more than one target disorder.

One way of approaching this is to sequentially estimate the post-test probability for multiple tests, by which the post-test probability after test A becomes the pre-test probability for test B. For example, in diagnosing deep venous thrombosis (DVT), the Wells' score (a series of clinical features found in patients with DVT) is often combined with the result of a blood test that measures how much blood clotting has occurred (D-dimer test). In a study of patients who were at high risk for developing DVT, the positive likelihood ratio (LR+) of the Wells' score alone was 21.4, which changed the pre-test probability of 16% to a post-test probability of 80%. Next, the results of the D-dimer test are applied. The D-dimer had an overall LR+ of 3.3, changing the new probability of 80% to 93% in patients testing positive.

This sequential computation of probabilities roughly corresponds to the actual probability of the combination of being at high risk on the Wells score *and* having a positive D-dimer test, which has an LR+ of 46, leading to a change in probability of 16% to 89% in that same study.

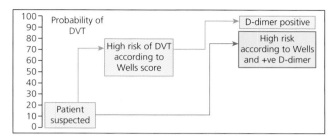

Figure 8.4

The sequential calculation of probabilities with LRs assumes that test A and test B are independent of each other. However, as we hinted earlier, this is not always the case.

For example, in children presenting to primary care with an acute illness, the probability of a serious infection when the parent is concerned changes from 1% to 12% (LR+ of 14). If, in addition to the parents' concern, the family doctor finds that the child is short of breath (LR+ of 9), the post-test probability increases from 12% to 55%. However, in reality the combination of parental concern and shortness of breath has an LR+ of 24, which changes the probability to only 20%.

This may come as no surprise, because the two tests are obviously not independent: the parents may be concerned precisely *because* their child has difficulty breathing. In other words, the diagnostic value of test A changes when test B is also used.

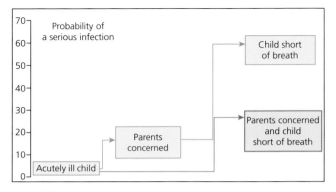

Figure 8.5

Multivariable analyses

There are several statistical techniques for analysing the diagnostic value of combinations of tests. With these techniques, the diagnostic value of each test is estimated while taking the value of the other tests into account. The end-product may be a list of signs and symptoms, a decision tree or a computerized algorithm.

To be useful in clinical practice, some criteria have to be met. First, the models need to be validated internally to avoid the use of over-optimistic (or over-fitted) models. Second, external validation is needed to test the robustness of the model, and to assess generalizability when it is applied in different populations. Finally, the rules or models need to be easy to implement in real-life clinical practice, where either the number of diagnostic variables is small or the model can be implemented using some sort of decision tool.

Logistic regression

This is the best-known technique, which calculates the adjusted odds ratio of multiple tests for one target disorder. Logistic regression is also used to build clinical prediction rules, in which scores (or weights) are assigned to the variables included in the model based on their coefficients.

Decision trees

These are a different type of multivariable analysis, in which tests are included sequentially to ultimately classify patients as having or not having the target disorder. Decision trees may also classify into more than two categories, i.e. including more than one target disorder.

Other techniques

More complicated techniques include latent class analysis and neural networks. Latent class analysis can be used when a true reference standard is absent. Neural networks are learning methods that model the presence or absence of the target disorder as a non-linear function of all available diagnostic information.

> **CLINICAL PREDICTION RULES**
> Clinical prediction rules are a common way of incorporating information from diagnostic studies into clinical practice. They bring together combinations of predictor variables, which may include clinical features as well as laboratory or imaging investigations. Clinical prediction rules attempt to simplify or streamline the diagnostic process, by identifying the clinical features that are the most useful (or predictive) for a particular outcome.

One popular clinical prediction rule is the Ottawa Ankle Rule (Figure 8.6). This was developed for patients presenting to the emergency department with acute ankle injuries, in order to help decide which ones need a radiograph of the ankle.

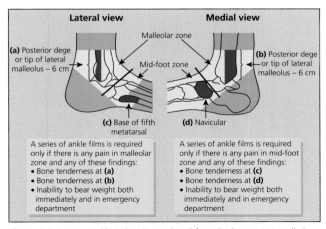

Lateral view   **Medial view**

Malleolar zone

(a) Posterior dege or tip of lateral malleolus – 6 cm

Mid-foot zone

(b) Posterior dege or tip of lateral malleolus – 6 cm

(c) Base of fifth metatarsal

(d) Navicular

A series of ankle films is required only if there is any pain in malleolar zone and any of these findings:
- Bone tenderness at **(a)**
- Bone tenderness at **(b)**
- Inability to bear weight both immediately and in emergency department

A series of ankle films is required only if there is any pain in mid-foot zone and any of these findings:
- Bone tenderness at **(c)**
- Bone tenderness at **(d)**
- Inability to bear weight both immediately and in emergency department

Figure 8.6 Ottawa Ankle Rules. (Reproduced from Bachmann LM, Kolb E, Koller MT, Steurer J, ter Riet G. Accuracy of Ottawa ankle rules to exclude fractures of the ankle and mid-foot: systematic review. *BMJ* 2003;**326**:417, with permission from BMJ Publishing Group Ltd.)

Clinical prediction rules can have a have a variety of potential uses in health care.

Uses of clinical prediction rules	Examples
The clinical decision is particularly complex	Prediction rule for identifying a child with a serious bacterial infection among the large number of children attending primary care with possible infection
Clinical outcome is rare and/or very serious	Prediction rule for risk of intracerebral bleed in child presenting with a minor non-penetrating head injury
To guide more invasive or costly investigations	Prediction rule for the need for knee radiograph in patients presenting to accident and emergency with acute knee trauma
As screening tests	The CAGE screening questionnaire to detect alcohol abuse
Determine prognosis	Framingham risk scores for cardiovascular disease
Teaching aids	An evidence-based way of approaching diagnosis can be a useful teaching aid for clinical trainees

How are clinical prediction rules developed?

There are three basic steps in developing and assessing the impact of prediction rules. It is important to be able to identify (and appraise) these steps in order to be able to determine how valuable and reliable a prediction rule may be in practice.

For many prediction rules these three steps will not all have been undertaken, and even if they have been they are unlikely to be found in the same research publication. In particular, few studies examine the impact of prediction rules.

Step 1: deriving clinical prediction rules

All the potentially important predictors that could possibly be associated with a given outcome of interest need to be identified. This might include all the features that would be obtained from taking a history, physical examination or the results of tests. Researchers identify a database from a large number of patients, some of whom have the outcome of interest, and make sure that all the clinical features are recorded. Ideally the clinicians or researchers who record or measure the predictors should not be the same ones who assess the outcome of interest. However, for many clinical settings this can be difficult to achieve.

Next, the clinical features that are most strongly associated with the outcome of interest are identified using one of several statistical techniques, such as logistic regression. This will yield a smaller number of predictors, which may vary in their relative importance (or weighting).

The predictive value of a newly derived clinical prediction rule can be assessed in several different ways. The simplest is its ability to discriminate people with and without the condition of interest. So measures such as sensitivity, specificity and LR may be quoted, all with appropriate confidence intervals to assess the certainty of the results. They can also be used to assign a categorical or numeric probability for a particular outcome (e.g. low, intermediate or high probability).

Step 2: validation

Validation is necessary because it is possible that predictors may have been associated with an outcome merely by chance. In addition, the population in which the rule was derived may be different from the population or setting in which others intend to apply it.

There are several statistical techniques that can be used to try to overcome the risk of chance associations. One is to split the derivation dataset into two parts, so that (for example) two-thirds of the data are used to derive the rule and the remaining third to validate it.

A more robust way is to explore how well the rule works when it is applied to different populations. This is important because the rule may perform well at a certain spectrum, severity, frequency of outcome, language, etc. – the more heterogeneous the validation populations (e.g. different hospitals, clinic systems, countries), the more robust the validation.

The quality of a validation study includes several of the issues that we outlined in Chapter 6, namely sequential recruitment of patients with appropriate spectrum, predictors measured/assessed accurately, assessors of outcome blind to presence of predictors, and sufficient numbers of patients in the validation study followed up for long enough to ensure that their disease status is definitively established.

Step 3: assess the impact

The aim of clinical prediction rules is to make an impact on patient outcomes. A clinical rule can be accurate and validated, yet have little or no impact on clinical care. This can occur if it is impractical, (e.g. it takes too much time, is too complicated), or if clinicians lack the skills or equipment needed to assess the necessary clinical variables to actually calculate the clinical prediction rule, or whether its safety has been assessed.

Determining the impact will vary depending on the rule, e.g. the impact of the Ottawa Ankle Rule on accident and emergency could be measured by the numbers of radiographs performed or avoided and a calculation of the resultant cost savings. It is usually impractical to randomize patients to have the clinical prediction rule applied. It is more common to use pre-/post-designs, where the impact of the rule is assessed before and after it is implemented.

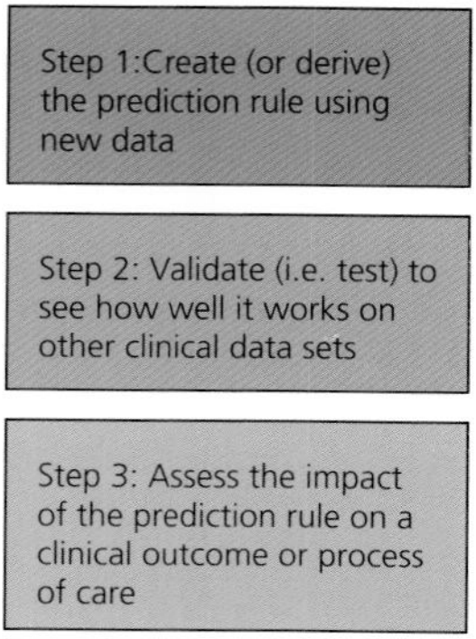

Step 1:Create (or derive) the prediction rule using new data

Step 2: Validate (i.e. test) to see how well it works on other clinical data sets

Step 3: Assess the impact of the prediction rule on a clinical outcome or process of care

Figure 8.7

How to select a prediction rule for clinical practice

Some clinical conditions have several prediction rules; in other conditions there may be only one (or none). Some of the important questions to ask when deciding whether to use a new prediction rule in a clinical setting include those in the table.

Selecting clinical prediction rules for clinical practice	
How valid is it?	Consider how the rule was derived and the level of validation in different populations or settings
How sensible is it?	Assessing whether a rule is likely to be sensible in clinical practice is a matter of clinical judgement. Predictors included in the model should be those that are (or can be) routinely collected, and measured in the same way. Some prediction rules may exclude predictors that clinicians currently use. A rule that does not include these may be less acceptable to clinicians
What is its potential impact?	Many studies of prediction rules compare how well the prediction rule performs with how well clinicians perform unaided by the rule. Although sensitivity or specificity may be better with the rule, clinical judgement may determine which of these are most important for the particular clinical situation. You may need to adjust the rule's cut-off point depending on whether it is most important to rule in or rule out the diagnosis. Ask yourself whether this decision is a limiting step in clinical practice anyway. How easy will it be to use it? How often is the rule likely to be overruled in clinical practice?

Based on Reilly BM, Evan AT. Translating clinical research into clinical practice: impact of using prediction rules to make decisions. *Ann Int Med* 2006;**144**:201–9.

Further reading

Beattie P, Nelson R. Clinical prediction rules: what are they and what do they tell us? *Aust J Physiother* 2006;**52**:157–63.

Brehaut JC, Stiell I, Graham I. Clinical decision rules 'in the real world': how a widely disseminated rule is used in everyday practice. *Acad Emerg Med* 2005;**12**:948–56.

Brehaut JC, Graham ID, Wood TJ, et al. Measuring acceptability of clinical decision rules: validation of the Ottawa acceptability of decision rules instrument (OADRI) in four countries. *Med Decis Making* 2010;**30**:398–408.

Heneghan C, Glasziou P, Thompson M, et al. Diagnostic strategies used in primary care. *BMJ* 2009;**338**:b946.

McGinn TG, Guyatt GH, Wyer PC, et al. Users' guides to the medical literature: XXII: how to use articles about clinical decision rules. Evidence-Based Medicine Working Group. *JAMA* 2000;**284**:79–84.

Reilly BM, Evans AT. Translating clinical research into clinical practice: impact of using prediction rules to make decisions. *Ann Intern Med* 2006;**144**:201–9.

CHAPTER 9
Screening tests

What are screening tests?

Screening involves using a test to identify a potential disease or target condition in people who are apparently well, i.e. they do not have (or do not recognize) any known signs or symptoms of that disease or condition. Screening tests aim to identify a disease or target condition earlier than the regular diagnostic process, which is initiated by a person feeling unwell or experiencing symptoms that cause distress or discomfort. By bringing forward the moment of diagnosis, the expectation is that interventions will be more effective, and mortality and morbidity will be reduced.

Different types of screening

- Screening for *unrecognized symptomatic disease*, i.e. screening for people who already have the disease that is causing them symptoms of which they are unaware (or have not reported to a clinician), e.g. screening for depression in elderly patients.
- Screening for *presymptomatic disease*, i.e. identifying people with disease that has not caused any symptoms yet, e.g. using faecal occult blood test to identify traces of blood in the stool of people with colon cancer.
- Screening for *risk factors*, i.e. identifying people who have risk factors for diseases that may occur some time in the future, e.g. measuring cholesterol levels in otherwise healthy individuals to identify those with lipid profiles, which places them a greater risk of future heart attacks.

In this sense, screening is a particular type of diagnostic testing, because it transforms some apparently well individuals into diseased individuals. The results of screening tests for unrecognized symptomatic or presymptomatic disease can be interpreted in the same way that we do for results of diagnostic tests (e.g. sensitivity, specificity), because the patients already have or do not have the disease of interest. For screening tests of risk factors, the element of time is important. Screening for risk factors involves predicting the new onset (i.e. incidence) of disease over a period of time (e.g. years).

The reason why screening tests or screening programmes need to be evaluated rigorously before they are implemented is because they can potentially cause problems as well as benefits.

Diagnostic Tests Toolkit, First Edition. Matthew Thompson, Ann Van den Bruel.
© 2012 John Wiley & Sons, Ltd. Published 2012 by John Wiley & Sons, Ltd.

Excessive screening can occur because:
- individuals like to think that prevention is better than cure
- most screening tests are applied to apparently healthy individuals, and there are often vast numbers (e.g. whole populations) of people eligible for screening tests
- encouragement from politicians, disease interest groups, manufacturers of tests and interventions.

Possible drawbacks of screening

	Drawback	Examples
Everyone	Pain, distress, anxiety, discomfort, side effects resulting from the actual screening test Cost of the test, time involved by the individual and health system	Some women find cervical screening unpleasant or uncomfortable Adopting a new screening programme might use health-care resources that could have been used for other patients.
False-negative screening test	Reassured incorrectly that they do not have the disease or risk factor	Failure of mammogram to identify a breast tumour due to poor quality reading
False- or true negative screening test	May take the reassurance as meaning that they are healthy in some other way, or change some other health behaviours	Normal BP reading taken in isolation by patients to imply that they are generally healthy
False-positive screening test	Anxiety and fear. Leads to additional diagnostic testing which can be unpleasant or have side effects	Raised PSA test leading to prostate biopsies, which subsequently are negative for prostate cancer
True positive screening test	Costs and treatment of the disease or risk factor may not be worth it The screening test detects a disease that would have remained unnoticed without screening ('over-diagnosis')	Prostatectomy for a very elderly man with positive prostate biopsy for an indolent cancer, causing urinary incontinence 'Over-diagnosis' might include a prostate cancer that remains indolent until the patient's death from another cause
False- or true positive screening test	Labelling, i.e. a positive result on a screening test might affect applications for employment, insurance, etc.	Positive screening test for hepatitis B active infection in a health-care worker

Deciding whether a screening programme is worthwhile

In 1968, Wilson and Jungner formulated principles of early disease detection that have been complemented by some more recent criteria to decide whether a screening programme is worthwhile (see box).

The condition must be an important health problem

There should be an accepted treatment for patients with recognized disease

Facilities for diagnosis and treatment should be available

There should be a recognizable latent or early symptomatic stage

There should be a suitable test or examination

The test should be acceptable to the population

The natural history of the condition should be adequately understood

There should be an agreed policy on whom to treat as patients

The costs should be economically balanced in relation to possible expenditure on medical care as a whole

Screening should be a continuous process and not a 'once and for all' project

Additional criteria (Dutch Health Council)

Treatment at an early stage is more beneficial than treatment at a later stage

The time between test and result should be as short as possible

Recruitment for participation may not impede people in their freedom to decide whether they will participate

Possible participants must receive information on benefit and harm of the screening programme

Public information must stress the universal access to the programme without exerting moral pressure to participate

Quality assurance and control of the programme has to be put in place

Screening programmes are concerted actions that require organization and management

---

Ideal study design for screening tests

The ideal study design to assess screening is a randomized study in which people are randomized into two groups (screened and not screened), and the total mortality is compared between the groups after a suitable period of time. By randomizing participants into the two groups, baseline differences should be evened out between the groups. By measuring total mortality we get away from the problem of cause-specific mortality (see below).

However, several different observational study designs can also be used to assess screening strategies. An observational study could use a comparison of the outcome (e.g. death from colon cancer) among people who happen to have been screened with those who have not been screened. Another type of observational study might look only at people who have the disease of interest, and compare screened patients with the disease with unscreened patients who also have that disease. Nevertheless, observational studies are more likely to give rise to biases than randomized trials.

WHAT ARE THE KEY BIASES IN SCREENING TESTS?
1. Volunteer (or selection bias)
2. Bias due to study type
3. Lead-time bias
4. Length–time bias

Volunteer (or selection) bias
People who participate in studies on screening differ from those who do not. Women at increased risk of breast cancer because of a family history may be more willing to participate in a screening trial, because of increased awareness of this disease. On the other hand, studies may require participants to travel to and from clinics, thereby excluding participants who are less mobile and possibly less healthy. These two examples show that selection may lead to the inclusion of participants who may be at both higher as well as lower risk of the target condition.

Bias due to study type
Observational studies that compare people undergoing screening to people not undergoing screening may find results that are attributable to differences in baseline risk rather than the effect of screening (confounding). Although randomized controlled trials may also suffer from selection bias due to differences in baseline risk of the study participants compared with the general population, the randomization ensures that the baseline risk is the same between the screened and the control groups.

This is illustrated in Figure 9.1. The green faces represent people at lower risk of the target condition and the red faces represent people at higher risk of the target condition. In the observational study, more healthy individuals tend to volunteer to be screened. This means that there are more people at lower risk who get screened, and more people at higher risk of the target condition who do not get screened. This can make the results of the study look better than they really are. In the randomized controlled trial, on the other hand, there are equal numbers of people with high and low risk in the screened and not-screened groups.

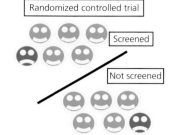

Figure 9.1

> TIP
> Randomized controlled trials are preferable to observational studies.

Lead-time bias

Most diseases have a period of time between the biological onset of the disease and when it causes symptoms. This is called the preclinical or 'latent' period. The main aim of screening is to try to identify or diagnose the disease in this latent period, before symptoms have occurred, and start treatment.

As screening brings forward the moment in time when diagnosis occurs, the time between diagnosis and death becomes longer even in situations where the moment of death has remained unchanged. This is called the *lead time*.

For example, a patient is screened and diagnosed with cancer at the age of 52. If he had not been screened, symptoms would have caused him to see a physician which would have led to a clinical diagnosis at the age of 59. However, in both cases, the patient dies at the age of 62.

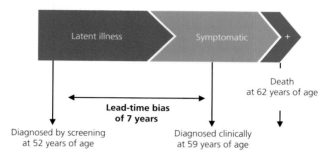

Figure 9.2

Seemingly, the patient's survival is better with screening (10 years) than without screening (3 years). In reality, *diagnosis was advanced* by 7 years. This is called *lead-time bias*. Lead-time bias affects a subgroup who will die of the condition whether or not they are screened and get treated. So, even if screening and treatment for that condition are not at all effective, counting the years of survival from the date of diagnosis can make the screened group *seem* like they are living longer.

> Beware of studies that measure a screening programme's success by *survival*. Survival is expressed as the number of people who died over a certain period from those diagnosed with the condition, whereas *mortality* is expressed as the number of people who died over a certain period (usually 1 year).

> **TIP**
> Look for studies that report mortality and survival.

Total mortality or disease-specific mortality

Ideally, you would like screening to reduce total mortality, because then people actually live longer. Accurate estimates of total mortality depend only on accurate recording of death, and not on recording what actually caused death. However, in most situations, the proportion of deaths caused by the disease that the screening programme is designed to detect is small compared with all other possible causes of death. Therefore, it is usually very difficult to show statistically significant effects on total mortality.

For these reasons, many screening studies report *disease-specific mortality* as the endpoint. This includes deaths caused by the target condition, treatment of the target condition and the screening test itself.

Misclassification may occur because patients screened and diagnosed with the target condition have more chance of receiving a disease-specific cause of death than patients not screened and not diagnosed with the target condition. This is called *sticky bias*.

Similarly, a patient who is not screened and not diagnosed with the target condition may still die of the target condition unnoticed. The effect of sticky bias is overestimation of the disease-specific mortality in the screened group, and under-estimation of the disease-specific mortality in the control group, thus leading to an under-estimation of the effect of screening.

An opposite cause of misclassification is *slippery bias*, where causes of death that are related to the screening and subsequent treatment are wrongly attributed to another cause. For example, a woman screened and diagnosed with breast cancer who then dies of heart failure after being treated with chemotherapy might be classified as having died of a non-breast cancer cause. The effect of slippery bias is under-estimation of the disease-specific mortality in the screened group.

Endpoint	Problems	Effect
Total mortality	Statistically significant effect difficult: proportion of deaths from target condition small in comparison with other causes of death	Too difficult to show that screening works
Disease-specific mortality	Sticky bias: once diagnosed with target condition, cause of death more easily attributed to target condition	Screening looks worse than it really is
	Slippery bias: cause of death is consequence of screening but is not recognized as such.	Screening looks better than it really is

Some studies find a decrease in disease-specific mortality but an increase in total mortality. This illustrates the difficulty in accurate recording of causes of death, and the possibility that screening in itself may cause harm and therefore increase total mortality.

> TIP
> Look at both all-cause mortality and disease-specific mortality.

Length–time bias

Many diseases are heterogeneous in the lengths of time people spend in the latent or presymptomatic phase of their illness. Typically there will be more rapidly progressive (aggressive) forms and more slowly progressive (indolent) forms of the disease.

People with the more rapidly progressive forms of the disease will have a shorter latent phase of their illness and will rapidly develop symptoms as the disease spreads. As a consequence, rapidly evolving forms of the condition will become symptomatic before screening, and the slowly evolving forms of the condition will remain asymptomatic until they are picked up by screening. Therefore, when screening for this condition, it is possible that the screening test will identify more people with the slowly progressive disease and fewer with the more aggressive disease.

This is also the reason why some patients may be diagnosed with the target condition shortly after participating in screening (in cancer, this is referred to as *interval cancers*). These patients may face a worse prognosis because this is more likely to be caused by a rapidly evolving form of the target condition.

This is illustrated in Figure 9.3, in which the first three patients have more rapidly developing or aggressive forms of the disease and develop symptoms before they have time to be screened ("wolves"). Let us say that they all live only a few years after diagnosis. The last three patients have slowly developing or less aggressive forms of the disease, and they are all identified by screening ("lambs"). Simply comparing the length of time survival between those screened and those not screened would tend to favour the screened group. However, this is simply because they have a less aggressive form of the disease which allowed them to be screened before symptoms develop and live longer after diagnosis.

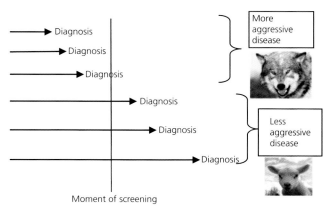

Figure 9.3

Over-diagnosis

This brings us to the problem of over-diagnosis (also called 'pseudo-disease'). Screening will diagnose the target condition in some patients who would otherwise never have had any symptoms during their lifetime. This can occur because the target condition is extremely slow in evolving, or because the person dies of another cause (e.g. a road traffic accident). These patients do not benefit from screening. On the contrary, they experience harm because they are diagnosed and potentially treated for a condition that they would not have been aware of without screening.

For example, a randomized trial used chest radiographs and sputum cytology to screen for lung cancer among 9211 male smokers in Minnesota (Marcus et al. 2000). The goal was that screening should identify lung tumours at an earlier stage and the unscreened group would have higher-grade lung tumours. After following the patients for a median of 20 years, there was a 29% increase in the cumulative incidence of lung tumours in the screened group, compared with the unscreened group. The screened group had earlier resectable lung tumours, but no decrease in late-stage tumours and lung cancer-related deaths. Why was this? Screening had picked up ('over-diagnosed') lots of low-grade early tumours that were not causing symptoms and probably would not go on to cause clinical disease.

In breast cancer, over-diagnosis as a result of screening is estimated at 29% (95% confidence interval [CI] 23–35). This means that, for every 100 women diagnosed with breast cancer clinically without screening, 129 women will be diagnosed with screening. Screening thus leads to 29 additional women diagnosed with breast cancer.

Further reading

Black WC. Overdiagnosis: An underrecognized cause of confusion and harm in cancer screening. *J Natl Cancer Inst* 2000;**92**:1280–2.

Grimes DA, Schulz KF. Uses and abuses of screening tests. *Lancet* 2002;**359**:881–4.

Marcus PM, Bergstralh EJ, Zweig MH, Harris A, Offord KP, Fontana RS. Extended lung cancer incidence follow-up in the Mayo Lung Project and overdiagnosis. *J Natl Cancer Inst* 2006;**98**:748–56.

Wilson JMG, Jungner G. *Principles and practice of screening for disease.* Public Health Papers no. 34. Geneva: WHO, 1968.

Yao SL, Lu-Yao G. Understanding and appreciating overdiagnosis in the PSA era. *J Natl Cancer Inst* 2002;**94**:958–60.

Gøtzsche PC, Nielsen M. Screening for breast cancer with mammography. *Cochrane Database Syst Rev.* 2011 Jan 19;(**1**):CD001877.

CHAPTER 10

Systematic reviews of diagnostic test accuracy studies

WHAT ARE THE KEY FEATURES OF SYSTEMATIC REVIEWS?
Systematic reviews of diagnostic test accuracy studies collate evidence and are designed to:
- identify and evaluate all of the existing research on a diagnostic test
- derive a more precise estimate of the diagnostic value of the test
- explore possible differences in value across different subgroups such as clinical setting.

This chapter describes the main steps when undertaking systematic reviews of diagnostic studies, and the key aspects to look out for when reading or assessing an existing review. The methods for doing systematic reviews of diagnostic studies are less established than those for interventions, and they can be more complicated to understand. The current trend seems to be for reviews that compare performance between diagnostic tests, rather than try to come up with a definitive accuracy estimate for one test (unlike systematic reviews and meta-analyses of intervention trials). We focus on systematic reviews of single diagnostic tests, rather than combinations of tests.

The research question

Identifying the relevant primary studies starts by structuring your research question. Use the same four elements that you used for finding diagnostic studies Chapter 3. These elements define the terms used when searching the electronic databases for primary studies to include in your systematic review.

Element	Specific example
Patient	Who are the patients?
Index test	Which test am I interested in?
Reference standard	What is the reference standard that is considered the best way of diagnosing the target condition?
Target condition	What is the target condition it should diagnose?

Diagnostic Tests Toolkit, First Edition. Matthew Thompson, Ann Van den Bruel.
© 2012 John Wiley & Sons, Ltd. Published 2012 by John Wiley & Sons, Ltd.

Systematic review research questions can be very *narrow* (e.g. 'What is the accuracy of dobutamine stress tests for the diagnosis of coronary artery disease in patients with chest pain?') or very *broad* (e.g. 'Which signs and symptoms are most accurate for the diagnosis of serious infections in children?'). However, a broad question is not the same as an unstructured question. All questions for a systematic review have to be structured and unambiguous. Broad research questions provide answers to many different aspects of the same clinical problem and can be more easily generalized to clinical practice. On the other hand, broad searches may provide such diverse results that it is difficult to summarize them in a meaningful way. If this is the case, consider splitting a broad question into several more narrow questions.

The literature search

Identify the available primary studies

Ideally, a systematic review compiles all the available evidence in a way that is reproducible. This usually means searching various databases complemented with other strategies such as reference tracking, expert consultation, hand-searching. Electronic databases that are mostly used are MedLine, EMBASE and DARE. Other databases include CINAHL, PEDRO, PsycLit and Medion. The choice of which database to use depends on the research question.

As mentioned in Chapter 4, search filters are often used to try to minimize the irrelevant studies, while not missing the studies that are most likely to be relevant to your search. For diagnostic systematic reviews it is important to use a sensitive search strategy, because diagnostic studies are often missed. This means combining thesaurus terms (e.g. MeSH terms in MedLine, EMTREE terms in EMBASE) with free text covering all possible synonyms. Beware, however, that a high yield does not necessarily mean that you have identified all relevant studies. If your terms are not well chosen, you may end up with lots of abstracts to read and still miss the most relevant studies.

> **EXAMPLE**
> Methods used to search in a systematic review of diagnostic symptoms and signs of children with serious infection in ambulatory care (Van den Bruel et al. 2010):
>
> We searched four electronic databases (Medline, Embase, DARE, and CINAHL). Search terms included MeSH terms and free text: 'serious infections', 'children', 'clinical and laboratory tests', and 'ambulatory care'. No time or language restrictions were placed on these searches. The first search was undertaken in October, 2008, with an update undertaken in

June, 2009. We checked reference lists of all retrieved articles and relevant guidelines from the National Institute for Health and Clinical Excellence published before 2008. The Medion database was checked for systematic reviews by use of the 'signs and symptoms' subheading. Additionally, domain experts were asked to review the list of studies identified and to report any obvious omissions.

Select the most relevant primary studies

Using the elements of your research question, the studies are then selected in two stages: first on title and abstract and, second, using their full text. Ideally the selection is done by two researchers independently, based on explicit criteria that may include other elements, e.g. design of the study. Piloting the selection process is recommended to limit the interrater variability and increase precision. Documenting the selection process using one of the widely available reference citation tools is the most convenient way to do this step.

EXAMPLE

Methods used to select studies in a systematic review of diagnostic symptoms and signs of children with serious infection in ambulatory care (Van den Bruel et al. 2010):

Selection was done by 2 independent reviewers, after piloting on a sample of 20 studies. Discrepancies between the reviewers were resolved by a 3rd independent reviewer. The studies were selected in 2 rounds, first on title and abstract and second on full text against 6 criteria:

Design: Studies that assessed diagnostic accuracy or derived prediction rules. We excluded narrative reviews, letters, editorials, comments and case series of <20 patients. Systematic reviews and meta analyses were used as source of references.

Participants: children 1month-18 years. Studies in children with immunosuppression were excluded.

Setting: ambulatory care settings in developed countries.

Outcome: serious infection, which included . . .

Diagnostic features: studies that assessed triage tests used in ambulatory care, including near patient tests. We excluded imaging, invasive tests, microbiological tests.

Data reporting: studies where construction of 2 × 2 tables were possible.

The process of selecting studies should be described, and it is best to display this with a flow chart, e.g. Figure 10.1.

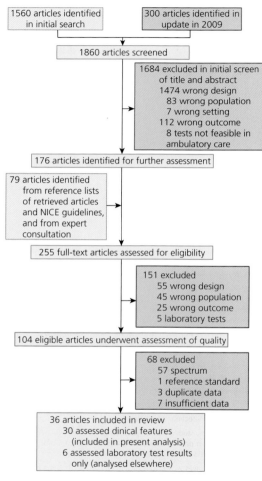

Figure 10.1

Assess the quality of individual studies included in the review

The most widely used scale for assessing the quality of individual diagnostic studies is QUADAS. It is based on empirical evidence on the design features that bias diagnostic accuracy results. Each item is scored with yes, no or unclear. It includes items related to internal validity of the study, as well as external validity. The items include all the sources of bias that were mentioned in Chapter 9 when appraising individual studies.

The QUADAS tool

1. Was the spectrum of patients representative of the patients who will receive the test in practice?

2. Were selection criteria clearly described?

3. Is the reference standard likely to correctly classify the target condition?

4. Is the time period between reference standard and index test short enough to be reasonably sure that the target condition did not change between the two tests?

5. Did the whole sample or a random selection of the sample receive verification using a reference standard of diagnosis?

6. Did patients receive the same reference standard regardless of the index test result?

7. Was the reference standard independent of the index test (i.e. the index test did not form part of the reference standard)?

8. Was the execution of the index test described in sufficient detail to permit replication of the test?

9. Was the execution of the reference standard described in sufficient detail to permit its replication?

10. Were the index test results interpreted without knowledge of the results of the reference standard?

11. Were the reference standard results interpreted without knowledge of the results of the index test?

12. Were the same clinical data available when test results were interpreted as would be available when the test is used in practice?

13. Were uninterpretable/intermediate test results reported?

14. Were withdrawals from the study explained?

From Whiting et al. (2003).

The interrater reliability of QUADAS has been shown to be moderate at best. Therefore it is important to have at least two reviewers assess the studies and resolve discrepancies by consensus or with a third independent reviewer. Also, it is worth remembering that studies may be assessed as being of poor quality either because they were conducted poorly or because they were reported poorly. The STAndards for Reporting of Diagnostic accuracy (STARD) initiative aims to improve the quality of reporting of studies of diagnostic accuracy. Many journals have adopted the STARD checklist for authors who are submitting manuscripts for publication (www.stard-statement.org).

Assessing the quality of studies included in diagnostic systematic reviews, even when using an explicit checklist such as QUADAS, remains subject to interpretation. Also, there is debate about the best ways of incorporating the results of quality assessment into systematic reviews.

Why assess quality?
There are several possible reasons why quality is assessed:
- 'Garbage in – garbage out', i.e. the results of a systematic review are totally dependent on the quality of the individual studies. A systematic review of poor quality studies cannot magically turn them into high-quality studies.
- As exclusion criteria, e.g. if the reference standard is deemed invalid (item 3 on the QUADAS list).
- To explore the sensitivity of the results to quality, i.e. whether diagnostic accuracy varies with the presence or absence of certain study features, e.g. analysis might consider the effect of whether the answer to item 11 on the QUADAS list (reference standard results interpreted blindly) were yes or no.
- To describe the quality of the primary studies included in the systematic review – often displayed using a table or bar charts for each item.

Extracting data
The results from each study are extracted, typically this will be a single 2×2 outcome for each study, but there may be several 2×2 tables from a single study. Usually the outcome is dichotomous, but predictors may be categorical or continuous. Typically the required information is extracted from the primary studies by one reviewer, and checked by a second reviewer. Errors that occur are discussed and corrected. Most researchers will use either a paper data extraction form or a spreadsheet to record the extracted information. The information extracted should also include characteristics of studies.

Summarizing the results of diagnostic studies
Summarizing the results of diagnostic studies is much more difficult than in systematic reviews of interventions for several reasons:
1. The results of diagnostic tests are two values, usually sensitivity and specificity (or positive and negative likelihood ratio [LR]), and it is not

possible to reduce this pair of numbers to a single value (such as a diagnostic odds ratio [OR]) without losing information. In addition, the values of sensitivity and specificity are dependent on each other, i.e. there is a trade-off so that when one is higher the other is lower (and vice versa).

2. The threshold (or cut-off) value used to define test results as positive or negative (or present or absent) often differs between studies (the 'threshold effect').

3. Diagnostic studies often have a lot of heterogeneity, i.e. they differ in their setting, study design, etc. – more so than primary studies of interventions.

Characteristics of the included studies

The primary studies that are included in the systematic review usually differ in some aspects. It is important to present the main characteristics of the included studies, because this may explain some of the differences (heterogeneity) in the results of the diagnostic test itself.

Some of the study characteristics that may be useful to present in a table include:

- design features (e.g. prospective/retrospective)
- recruitment strategy (e.g. consecutive/case–control)
- setting (e.g. country, type of health-care setting, i.e. primary care/ secondary care)
- participants (e.g. inclusion and exclusion criteria, age, gender, ethnicity, numbers with and without disease)
- details on the index test (e.g. how was it done, thresholds of cut-offs used)
- details of the reference standard (this may vary between different studies)
- target condition (e.g. prevalence, severity).

Presenting the results of the individual studies

There are several different ways to graphically present the data on diagnostic accuracy from individual studies. These can be very informative and are one way of looking for differences in results (i.e. heterogeneity) between studies or across subgroups of patients or studies. Sometimes the interpretation of the heterogeneity observed can be one of the most useful parts of a diagnostic systematic review.

The simplest way of presenting these is to list sensitivity and specificity (and other diagnostic accuracy measures) from each study in a table.

Forest plot

A Forest plot can present all the individual pairs of sensitivity and specificity (or LRs), along with their confidence intervals. Sometimes the numerators and denominators can be included. This often demonstrates the co-variation between pairs of sensitivity and specificity (i.e. as one gets bigger, the other gets smaller).

EXAMPLE
C-reactive protein for the diagnosis of serious infections in children.

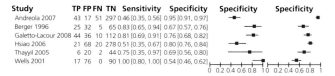

Study	TP	FP	FN	TN	Sensitivity	Specificity
Andreola 2007	43	17	51	297	0.46 [0.35, 0.56]	0.95 [0.91, 0.97]
Berger 1996	25	32	5	65	0.83 [0.65, 0.94]	0.67 [0.57, 0.76]
Galetto-Lacour 2008	44	36	10	112	0.81 [0.69, 0.91]	0.76 [0.68, 0.82]
Hsiao 2006	21	68	20	278	0.51 [0.35, 0.67]	0.80 [0.76, 0.84]
Thayyil 2005	6	20	2	44	0.75 [0.35, 0.97]	0.69 [0.56, 0.80]
Wells 2001	17	76	0	90	1.00 [0.80, 1.00]	0.54 [0.46, 0.62]

Figure 10.2

Presenting sensitivity and 1 – specificity pairs on an ROC plot
The individual pairs of sensitivity and 1 – specificity from individual studies
can be plotted on a receiver operating characteristics (ROC) curve. Looking
at the scatter of the point estimates of sensitivity and 1 – specificity gives
some information about the overall performance of the test. It also lets you
see how much variation there is between studies, which may be for many
different reasons: random variation between studies, heterogeneity in study
designs, different thresholds, etc. In fact this variation is what makes this
type of simple summary curve so difficult to interpret; you simply cannot tell
what is causing difference between studies (Figure 10.3).

Using the same data that we displayed above using a Forest plot, the ROC
in Figure 10.3 below shows the sensitivity and specificity of C-reactive
protein (CRP) for the diagnosis of serious infections in children.

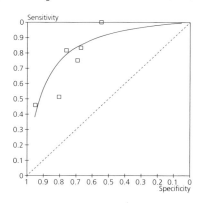

Figure 10.3

Scatter plots

To show a possible relationship between the diagnostic value of the
index test and another variable, e.g. prevalence or cut-off value, a
simple scatter plot of the outcome measure of interest and the variable
of interest can be very informative. Figure 10.4 is an example of a scatter
plot of the likelihood ratios (LR+ in red and LR– in blue) of coronary
angiography for coronary artery disease reported in over 30 studies,
plotted against the prevalence of coronary artery disease from the original
study. It suggests that, as prevalence increases, both LR+ and LR– decrease
and, as such, coronary angiography is more suitable to rule in in a low-
prevalence setting and more suitable to rule out in a high-prevalence setting.
This example is taken from a systematic review, but a similar plot may be
useful in primary studies reporting different cut-offs or different patient
subgroups.

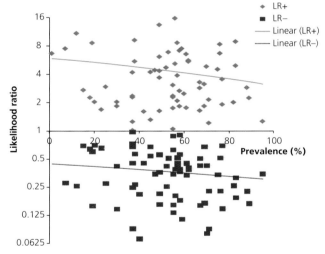

Figure 10.4

Dumbbell plots

Dumbbell plots show how the pre-test probability (or prevalence) changes
after a positive or negative index test. The pre-test probability is displayed
with a blue dot, the post-test probability after a positive test with a red dot

and the post-test probability after a negative test with a green dot.
Dumbbell plots can be used to present the results of primary studies, to
show results on subgroups or different index tests, or in systematic reviews
to present the results of the different studies.

Study	Setting	Cut-off used	Likelihood ratios		Probability of illness		
			LR+	LR−	Before test ●	After test if + ○	After test if− ○
Index test 1							
Study a	Int	prolonged	2.05 (1.01-4.19)	0.87 (0.72-1.04)			
Study b	Int	≥1.18	13.1 (1.23-38.8)	0.92 (0.82-1.04)			
Index test 2							
Study b	Int	≥1.2	13.1 (5.88-29.0)	0.44 (0.27-0.70)			
Index test 3		**(1000/mm³)**					
Study b	Int	≤150	3.20 (1.36-7.53)	0.81 (0.64-1.03)			

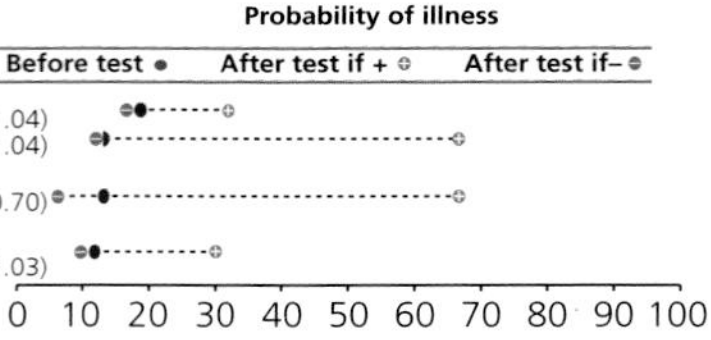

0 10 20 30 40 50 60 70 80 90 100

Figure 10.5

Post-test versus pre-test probability plots

These are an alternative to the dumbbell plots and present the change in
probability for a positive and a negative test result, depending on the
pre-test probability. The main advantages of these plots are that they can
present more than one result, and they can be used to explore the
relationship between prevalence and post-test probability.

Another useful feature of this plot is that it can show the asymmetry of a
test, because the change in probability may be quite different for positive
and negative tests. This plot can be particularly useful for displaying the
results of systematic reviews that identify studies in different settings with
different prevalences (i.e. different pre-test probabilities).

Figure 10.6 shows the results of a systematic review that explores the
change in probability of serious infection in children based on their
temperature level (fever). The triangles represent studies using cut-offs of
38.5°C, circles represent studies using temperature cut-offs of 39°C and
squares are cut-offs of 40°C. Figure 10.6 shows the change in probability of
a serious infection, depending on whether the child's temperature is above
(solid symbol) or below (open symbol) that threshold. The diagonal line
represents a study where the pre- and post-test probabilities are the same
(i.e. the test has no value). For example, the first symbol on the left is a
square, i.e. that study used a temperature cut-off of ≥40°C. In that particular
study, the pre-test probability of serious infection was 0.78%. If the child
had a temperature of ≥40°C, then the probability of a serious infection
increases to 5%. If the child did not have a temperature of ≥40°C, then the
probability remains at more or less the same level.

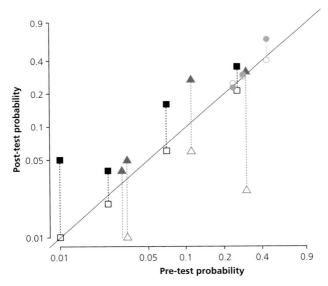

Figure 10.6

Combining data and interpreting meta-analyses of diagnostic studies

Before looking at the results of a meta-analysis, always consider whether it makes sense to combine diagnostic accuracy data in this way. Meta-analysis may be inappropriate when the individual studies are too heterogeneous, or of poor quality, because the results may potentially be misleading.

If the studies are heterogeneous, it is worth exploring whether study characteristics potentially explain some of the observed variation between studies. If meta-analysis is not possible, a diagnostic systematic review is still useful, and is usually presented as a descriptive analysis of the available evidence from which conclusions can be drawn – using the graphs that we described above.

There are more formal ways of assessing heterogeneity, some of which are quite complicated. When Forest plots are used to present the findings, a simple method to examine heterogeneity is to look at the overlap of the confidence intervals.

Meta-analyses are a way of estimating 'an average' or 'common' effect. This can give a more precise estimate of the diagnostic value of a test because it pools all available data from several studies. There are several mathematical ways of doing this for diagnostic systematic reviews.

Simply pooling together sensitivity or specificity gives an estimate of this 'average' effect. However, it is too simplistic because it ignores some of the details of diagnostic accuracy studies such as different thresholds or heterogeneity between studies, as well as the correlation between sensitivity and specificity.

For example, in a meta-analysis of three studies that had markedly different values of sensitivity and specificity, namely study 1 10% and 90%, study 2 80% and 80% and study 3 90% and 10%. Simply averaging these would give sensitivity of 60% and specificity of 60% – which does not really tell us anything useful about these data!

Moses Littenberg summary ROC curve

This method of meta-analysis models the association between the logarithm of the diagnostic OR and a measure of diagnostic threshold used for each study using simple linear regression. This method accounts for the correlation between sensitivity and specificity, but is not thought to be statistically rigorous because it ignores some of the assumptions that are important for linear regression (constant variance and co-variate measured without error) and does not provide estimates of the heterogeneity between studies.

Hierarchical summary ROC curves and bivariate random effects models

If the individual studies are sufficiently homogeneous, there are two more advanced mathematical models that are now accepted as statistically valid when pooling results of studies in diagnostic systematic reviews: (1) hierarchical summary ROC curves and (2) the bivariate random effects model. Both of these models incorporate the variation between studies (both use random effects) to give a summary ROC curve or an 'average' sensitivity and specificity. Even more complex methods can be used when there is more than one possible threshold value (e.g. see Dukic and Gatsonis 2006; Hamza et al. 2009). These all require specialized statistical software and expertise.

Hierarchical summary ROC curves use the relationship between log-transformed sensitivity and specificity which is expressed in terms of the diagnostic OR and threshold. It assumes an explicit formula linking sensitivity and specificity throughout a threshold to provide estimates for this association that will help summarize it as a summary ROC curve.

The bivariate random effects model is based on jointly modelling the sensitivity and specificity while including the correlation between them and incorporating some of the unexplained variation in these parameters (random effects). It produces estimates of the average sensitivity and specificity and provides a confidence region (two dimensions) for this summary point.

Figure 10.7 shows a plot of individual values of test accuracy of a treadmill echocardiogram for coronary artery disease obtained from 11 studies. Each study is represented by a circle. The size of each circle is proportional to the numbers of patients in the study. A summary ROC is superimposed using a hierarchical ROC model, whereas a 95% confidence region and a 95% prediction region were estimated using a bivariate random effects model.

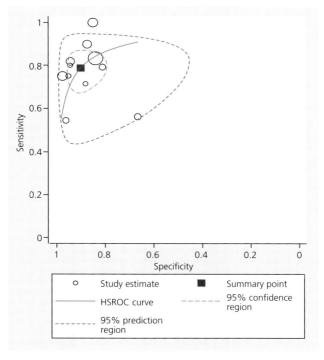

Figure 10.7

Interpreting/applying the overall results of a diagnostic systematic review

Diagnostic systematic reviews are not academic exercises; they are valuable only if their results are applied to real health-care problems. Assuming that the systematic review meets the objectives of the study question and that the search process and methodology were robust, the results should be interpreted with these questions in mind:

- How likely are the results to be biased?
- What effects did differences in quality between studies probably have on the results?
- How do the data provide information about how a test should be used, particularly in comparison to other (existing) tests?
- What are the clinical consequences of false-positive and false-negative results?
- Can the results of the systematic review be used to influence at the health-care policy level, for example, which diagnostic test to recommend?
- How close are the included studies to the intended future role of the test?
- If more primary studies are needed, what are the key questions that still need to be answered and what are the main quality areas that should be improved?

Reporting diagnostic systematic reviews

The PRISMA statement offers guidelines for authors who wish to report systematic reviews and meta-analyses. The PRISMA statement is available from www.prisma-statement.org.

Acknowledgements

Several figures and excerpts in this chapter have been reprinted from Van den Bruel et al. (2010), with permission from Elsevier.

Further reading

Devillé WL, Buntinx F, Bouter LM, et al. Conducting systematic reviews of diagnostic studies: didactic guidelines. *BMC Med Res Methodol* 2002;**2**:9.

Dukic V, Gatsonis C. Meta-analysis of diagnostic test accuracy assessment studies with varying number of thresholds. *Biometrics* 2003;**59**:936–46.

Hamza TH, Arends LR, van Houwelingen HC, Stijnen T. Multivariate random effects meta-analysis of diagnostic tests with multiple thresholds. *BMC Med Res Methodol* 2009;**9**:73.

Gatsonis C, Paliwal P. Meta-analysis of diagnostic and screening test accuracy evaluations: methodologic primer. *AJR Am J Roentgenol* 2006;**187**:271–81.

Harbord RM, Deeks JJ, Egger M, Whiting P, Sterne JA. A unification of models for meta-analysis of diagnostic accuracy studies. *Biostatistics* **2007**;8:239–51. Erratum: *Biostatistics* 2008;**9**:779.

Leeflang MM, Deeks JJ, Gatsonis C, Bossuyt PM, Cochrane Diagnostic Test Accuracy Working Group. Systematic reviews of diagnostic test accuracy. *Ann Intern Med* 2008;**149**:889–97.

Van den Bruel A, Haj-Hassan T, Thompson M, Buntinx F, Mant D. Diagnostic value of clinical features at presentation to identify serious infection in children in developed countries: a systematic review. *Lancet* 2010;**375**:834–45.

Whiting P, Rutjes AW, Reitsma JB, Bossuyt PM, Kleijnen J. The development of QUADAS: a tool for the quality assessment of studies of diagnostic accuracy included in systematic reviews. *BMC Med Res Methodol* 2003;**3**:25

Whiting P, Harbord R, de Salis I, Egger M, Sterne J. Evidence-based diagnosis. *J Health Serv Res Policy* 2008;**13**(suppl 3):57–63.

APPENDIX 1

Evidence-based medicine – a glossary of terms

http://www.cebm.net

Adjustment: a summarizing procedure for a statistical measure in which the effects of differences in composition of the populations being compared have been minimized by statistical methods.

Analytical variability: this affects the reproducibility of a test, and consists of inaccuracy, which is a systematic error, and imprecision, which is a random error.

Association: statistical dependence between two or more events, characteristics or other variables. An association may be fortuitous or produced by various other circumstances; the presence of an association does not necessarily imply a causal relationship.

Bias: any tendency to influence the results of a trial (or their interpretation) other than the experimental intervention.

Blinding: a technique used in research to eliminate bias by hiding the intervention from the patient, clinician and/or other researchers who are interpreting results.

Blind(ed) study (masked study): a study in which observer(s) and/or participants are kept ignorant of the group to which the participants are assigned, as in an experimental study, or of the population from which the participants come, as in a non-experimental or observational study.

Blobbogram: see Forest plot.

Case–control study: involves identifying patients who have the outcome of interest (cases) and control patients without the same outcome, and performing the index test to analyse its accuracy.

Case-series: a report on a series of patients with an outcome of interest. No control group is involved.

Clinical practice guideline: a systematically developed statement designed to help health-care professionals and patients make decisions about appropriate health care for specific clinical circumstances.

Clinical prediction rules: a combination of clinical predictors (e.g. clinical features, laboratory tests) that are the most useful (or predictive) for a particular outcome.

Cochrane Collaboration: a worldwide association of groups that create and maintain systematic reviews for specific topic areas.

Diagnostic Tests Toolkit, First Edition. Matthew Thompson, Ann Van den Bruel.
© 2012 John Wiley & Sons, Ltd. Published 2012 by John Wiley & Sons, Ltd.

Coding: the assignment of (usually numeric) codes to each category of each variable.

Cohort study: involves the identification of one or more groups (cohorts) of patients, who share some characteristic of interest.

Co-morbidity: coexistence of a disease or diseases in a study participant in addition to the index condition that is the subject of study.

Comparison group: any group to which the intervention group is compared. Usually synonymous with control group.

Confidence interval (CI): the range around a study's result within which we would expect the true value to lie. CIs account for the sampling error between the study population and the wider population that the study is supposed to represent.

Confounding variable: a variable that is not the one in which you are interested but that may affect the results of trial.

Cost–benefit analysis: economic evaluation in which all costs and consequences of a health intervention are expressed in the same units, usually money.

Cost-effectiveness analysis: economic evaluation in which the costs and consequences of alternative interventions are expressed as cost per unit of health outcome.

Cost–utility analysis: economic study design in which interventions which produce different consequences, in terms of both quantity and quality of life, are expressed as 'utilities' (e.g. cost per additional QUALY). See Utility.

Critically appraised topic (CAT): a short summary of an article from the literature, created to answer a specific clinical question.

Cross-sectional study: a study that observes a defined population at a single point in time or time interval. Exposure and outcome are determined simultaneously.

Determinant: any definable factor that effects a change in a health condition or other characteristic.

Diagnostic odds ratio: diagnostic odds ratio (DOR) is the odds for a positive test result in diseased people relative to the odds of a positive result in non-diseased people.

Differential reference bias: bias caused by the application of one reference standard in some patients and another reference standard in the remaining patients.

Dumbbell plots: graphic plots that display the change in probability of illness depending on a positive or negative index test result.

Effectiveness: a measure of the benefit resulting from an intervention for a given health problem under the usual conditions of clinical care for a particular group.

Efficacy: a measure of the benefit resulting from an intervention for a given health problem under the ideal conditions of a research study.

Evidence-based health care: the application of the principles of evidence-based medicine (see below) to all professions associated with health care, including purchasing and management.

Evidence-based medicine: the conscientious, explicit and judicious use of current best evidence in making decisions about the care of individual patients. The practice of evidence-based medicine means integrating individual clinical expertise with the best available external clinical evidence from systematic research.

Exclusion criteria: conditions that preclude entrance of candidates into an investigation even if they meet the inclusion criteria.

External validity: relates to the generalizability of a study.

Face validity: assesses if the test is a reasonable tool for the condition.

Fixed effects model: statistical method for pooling the results of different studies, assuming that there is only one true underlying effect and all differences between studies are due to chance.

Follow up: observation over a period of time of an individual, group or initially defined population whose relevant characteristics have been assessed in order to observe changes in health status or health-related variables.

Forest plot: a diagrammatic representation of the results of individual trials in a meta-analysis.

Gold standard: see Reference standard.

Hazard ratio: reflects the analysis of time survived to an event.

Heterogeneity: in systematic reviews, the amount of incompatibility between trials included in the review, whether clinical (i.e. the studies are clinically different) or statistical (i.e. the results are different from one another).

Incidence: the number of new cases of illness commencing, or of people falling ill, during a specified time period in a given population.

Incorporation bias: when the index test is a part of the reference standard, or vice versa.

Index test: the index test is the test that you want to study or analyse.

Internal validity: refers to whether the study is free from bias.

Lead-time bias: if prognosis study patients are not all enrolled at similar, well-defined points in the course of their disease, differences in outcome over time may merely reflect differences in duration of illness.

Length–time bias: bias that can distort the results of studies on screening tests, because slow-growing tumours (which have a better prognosis) are more likely to be picked up by screening than fast-growing tumours.

Likelihood ratio (LR): the likelihood that a given test result would be expected in a patient with the target disorder compared with the likelihood that the same result would be expected in a patient without that disorder.

Linear regression: statistical approach to model the relationship between a variable *y* and one or more variables *x*.

Logistic regression: statistical approach to predict the probability of a dichotomous outcome based on several predictors.

MeSH: Medical Subject Headings: a thesaurus of medical terms used by many databases and libraries to index and classify medical information.

Meta-analysis: a systematic review that uses quantitative methods to summarise the results.

Morbidity: diseased state, disability or poor health due to any cause

Negative predictive value (NPV): the proportion of people with a negative test who are free of disease.

Nested case–control study: case–control study in which all participants are samples from the same reference population.

Observer bias: bias in a trial where the measurement of outcomes or disease severity may be subject to bias because observers are not blinded to the patients' treatment.

Observer variation: this consists of interobserver variation (more than one observer interprets the same test, and assesses the extent to which they agree or disagree about the result) and intraobserver variation (the same observer interprets the same test on more than one occasion).

Odds: a ratio of events to non-events. If the event rate for a disease is 0.1 (10%), its non-event rate is 0.9 and therefore its odds are 1/9.

Overview: a summary of medical literature in a particular area.

P value: the probability that a particular result would have happened by chance.

Paired study: diagnostic accuracy study in which all participants undergo two index tests and the reference standard

Positive predictive value (PPV): the proportion of people with a positive test who have the outcome of interest.

Post-test probability: the probability that a patient has the disorder of interest after the test result is known.

Pre- and post-designs: also referred to as before–after designs: comparison of outcome (i.e. diagnosis) before and after the introduction of a new diagnostic test or strategy.

Pre-test probability: the probability that a patient has the disorder of interest before administering a test.

Prevalence: the baseline risk of a disorder in the population of interest.

PRISMA: statement on the reporting of systematic reviews.

Prospective study: study design where one or more groups (**cohorts**) of individuals who have not yet had the outcome event in question are monitored for the number of such events that occur over time.

Publication bias: a bias in a systematic review caused by incompleteness of the search, such as omitting non-English language sources or unpublished trials (inconclusive trials are less likely to be published than conclusive ones, but are not necessarily less valid).

QALY: quality-adjusted life-year.

QUADAS: tool for the quality assessment of studies of diagnostic accuracy included in systematic reviews.

Random effects model: statistical model for pooling the results of different studies that assumes that the differences in effect between the studies are due to chance and to true variation. It assumes the existence of a population of possible effects distributed around a mean overall effect.

Randomized controlled clinical trial: a group of patients is randomized into an experimental group and a control group. These groups are followed up for the variables/outcomes of interest.

Recall bias: systematic error due to the differences in accuracy or completeness of recall to memory of past events or experiences.

Receiver operator characteristics (ROC) curve: graphic plot of the sensitivity and 1 − specificity.

Reference standard: a diagnostic test (also called 'gold standard') used in trials to confirm the presence or absence of the target disorder.

Referral filter bias: the sequence of referrals that may lead patients from primary to tertiary centres raises the proportion of more severe or unusual cases, thus increasing the likelihood of adverse or unfavourable outcomes.

Reproducibility (repeatability, reliability): the results of a test or measure are identical or closely similar each time that it is conducted. Reproducibility depends on analytical variability and observer variation.

Retrospective study: study design in which cases where individuals who had an outcome event in question are collected and analysed after the outcomes have occurred.

Risk: the probability that an event will occur for a particular patient or group of patients. Risk can be expressed as a decimal fraction or percentage (0.25 = 25%).

Scatter plots: graphic plot of two variables.

Selection bias: a bias in assignment or selection of patients for a study that arises from study design rather than by chance. This can occur when the study and control groups are chosen so that they differ from each other by one or more factors that may affect the outcome of the study.

Sensitivity: the proportion of people with disease who have a positive test.

Sensitivity analysis: a process of testing how sensitive a result would be to changes in factors such as baseline risk, susceptibility, and the patients' best and worst outcomes, etc.

Slippery bias: where deaths due to diagnostic or therapeutic interventions that are a result of screening are not included in disease-specific mortality.

SnNout: when a test has a high sensitivity, a negative result rules out the diagnosis.

Specificity: the proportion of people free of a disease who have a negative test.

Spectrum bias: a bias caused by a study population whose disease profile does not reflect that of the intended population (e.g. if they have more severe forms of the disorder).

SpPin: when a test has a high specificity, a positive result rules in the diagnosis.

STARD: STAndards for the Reporting of Diagnostic accuracy studies.

Sticky bias: where deaths from other causes in the screened group are wrongly attributed to the target cancer or deaths in the control group are wrongly attributed to other causes.

Stratification: division into groups. Stratification may also refer to a process to control for differences in confounding variables, by making separate estimates for groups of individuals who have the same values for the confounding variable.

Survival: proportion of patients alive at some point subsequent to the diagnosis of their illness.

Systematic review: an article in which the authors have systematically searched for, appraised and summarized all of the medical literature for a specific topic.

Validity: the extent to which a variable or intervention measures what it is supposed to measure or accomplishes what it is supposed to accomplish. The **internal validity** of a study refers to the integrity of the experimental design. The **external validity** of a study refers to the appropriateness by which its results can be applied or generalized to non-study patients or populations.

Youden index: is calculated as (sensitivity + specificity) − 1. For a test to be useful, the Youden index should be greater than zero, e.g. flipping a coin with heads meaning positive and tails negative, the sensitivity and specificity will both be 0.5, giving a Youden index of zero, i.e. not useful.

APPENDIX 2
Further reading

Books
Heneghan C, Badenoch D. *Evidence-based Medicine Toolkit*, 2nd edn. London: Blackwell Publishing, 2006.
Hulley SB, ed. *Designing Clinical Research: An epidemiologic approach*, 2nd edn. Philadelphia: Lippincott Williams & Wilkins, 2001.
Knottnerus JA, Buntinx F, eds. *The Evidence Base of Clinical Diagnosis – Theory and methods of diagnostic research*. 2nd edn. London: Blackwell Publishing, 2009.
McGee S. *Evidence Based Physical Diagnosis*, 2nd edn. Philadelphia: Saunders, 2007.
Newman T, John M. *Evidence-based Diagnosis*. Cambridge: Cambridge Medicine, 2009.
Polmear A. *Evidence-based Diagnosis in Primary Care*. Oxford: Butterworth Heinemann, 2007.
Price C, ed. *Applying Evidence-based Laboratory Medicine: A step-by-step guide*. Washington DC: AACC Press, 2009.
Simel D, Rennie D. *The Rational Clinical Examination: Evidence-based clinical diagnosis*. JAMA & Archives Journals, 2006. McGraw-Hill e-books, copyright by the American Medical Association, ISBN 0071590307.
Steyerberg EW. *Clinical Prediction Models. A practical approach to development, validation, and updating*. New York: Springer, 2009.
Summerton N. *Patient-centred Diagnosis*. Oxford: Radcliffe Publishing, 2007.

Useful websites
www.effectivehealthcare.ahrq.gov: Agency for Healthcare Research and Quality (AHRQ) Methods Guide for Medical Test reviews (available freely).
www.stard-statement.org: Standards for Reporting of Diagnostic Accuracy (STARD) initiative aims to improve the quality of reporting of studies of diagnostic accuracy. Many journals have adopted the STARD checklist for authors who are submitting manuscripts for publication.

Useful journal articles
Elstein AS, Schwartz A. Clinical problem solving and diagnostic decision making: selective review of the cognitive literature. *BMJ* 2002;**32–4**:729–32 (review of the literature on how clinicians make diagnostic decisions).
Feinstein A. Misguided efforts and future challenges for research on 'diagnostic tests'. *J Epidemiol Commun Health* 2002;**56**:330–2 (suggests some of the current methods used to evaluate markers are not satisfactory).
Fryback DG, Thornbury JR. The efficacy of diagnostic imaging. *Med Decis Making* 1991;**11**:88–94 (a classic article on the stages in assessing diagnostic studies).
Glasziou P, Irwig L, Deeks J. When should a new test become the current reference standard? *Ann Intern Med* 2008;**149**:816–21 (sometimes a new diagnostic test can be better than the 'gold standard'; this gives some examples of what to do).

Diagnostic Tests Toolkit, First Edition. Matthew Thompson, Ann Van den Bruel.
© 2012 John Wiley & Sons, Ltd. Published 2012 by John Wiley & Sons, Ltd.

Grimes DA, Schulz KF. Refining clinical diagnosis with likelihood ratios. *Lancet* 2005;**365**:1500–5 (one of a series of excellent articles in the Lancet on epidemiology).

Reid MC, Lane DA, Feinstein AR. Academic calculations versus clinical judgments: practicing physicians' use of quantitative measures of test accuracy. *Am J Med* 1998;**104**:374–80 (describes the result of a survey which highlighted the difficulties that clinicians have using numeric measures of test accuracy).

Whiting PF, Sterne JA, Westwood ME, et al. Graphical presentation of diagnostic information. *BMC Med Res Methodol* 2008;8:20 (provides description and examples of the different graphs you can use to display results of diagnostic test results).

Index

STARD checklist for reporting studies of diagnostic accuracy. Reproduced by permission of STARD.

Please refer to www.stard-statement.org for a more detailed discussion and examples of the checklist items

Section and Topic	Item no.		On page no.
Title/Abstract/ Keywords	1	Identify the article as a study of diagnostic accuracy (recommend MeSH heading 'sensitivity and specificity')	
Introduction	2	State the research questions or study aims, such as estimating diagnostic accuracy or comparing accuracy between tests or across participant groups	
Methods *Participants*	3	The study population: The inclusion and exclusion criteria, setting and locations where data were collected	
	4	Participant recruitment: Was recruitment based on presenting symptoms, results from previous tests, or the fact that the participants had received the index tests or the reference standard?	
	5	Participant sampling: Was the study population a consecutive series of participants defined by the selection criteria in item 3 and 4? If not, specify how participants were further selected	
	6	Data collection: Was data collection planned before the index test and reference standard were performed (prospective study) or after (retrospective study)?	
Test methods	7	The reference standard and its rationale	
	8	Technical specifications of material and methods involved including how and when measurements were taken, and/or cite references for index tests and reference standard	
	9	Definition of and rationale for the units, cut-offs and/or categories of the results of the index tests and the reference standard	
	10	The number, training and expertise of the persons executing and reading the index tests and the reference standard	
	11	Whether or not the readers of the index tests and reference standard were blind (masked) to the results of the other test and describe any other clinical information available to the readers	